Atlas of
Minimally Invasive Surgical Techniques

Atlas of
Minimally Invasive Surgical Techniques

Editors:

Ashley H. Vernon, MD
Associate Surgeon
Division of General and Gastrointestinal Surgery
Brigham and Women's Hospital
Boston, Massachusetts

Stanley W. Ashley, MD
Chief Medical Officer Brigham and Women's Hospital Frank Sawyer Professor of Surgery Harvard Medical School
Boston, Massachusetts

Series Editors:

Courtney M.Townsend, Jr., MD
Professor and John Woods Harris Distinguished Chairman
Robertson-Poth Distinguished Chair in General Surgery
Department of Surgery
The University of Texas Medical Branch
Galveston, Texas

B. Mark Evers, MD
Professor and Vice-Chair for Research
Department of Surgery
Markey Cancer Foundation Endowed Chair
Director, Markey Cancer Center
University of Kentucky
Lexington, Kentucky

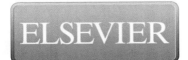

3251 Riverport Lane
St. Louis, Missouri 63043

ATLAS OF MINIMALLY INVASIVE SURGICAL TECHNIQUES

ISBN: 978-1416046967

Notices

Knowledge and best practice in this field are constantly changing. As new research and experience broaden our understanding, changes in research methods, professional practices, or medical treatment may become necessary.

Practitioners and researchers must always rely on their own experience and knowledge in evaluating and using any information, methods, compounds, or experiments described herein. In using such information or methods they should be mindful of their own safety and the safety of others, including parties for whom they have a professional responsibility.

With respect to any drug or pharmaceutical products identified, readers are advised to check the most current information provided (i) on procedures featured or (ii) by the manufacturer of each product to be administered, to verify the recommended dose or formula, the method and duration of administration, and contraindications. It is the responsibility of practitioners, relying on their own experience and knowledge of their patients, to make diagnoses, to determine dosages and the best treatment for each individual patient, and to take all appropriate safety precautions.

To the fullest extent of the law, neither the Publisher nor the authors, contributors, or editors, assume any liability for any injury and/or damage to persons or property as a matter of products liability, negligence or otherwise, or from any use or operation of any methods, products, instructions, or ideas contained in the material herein.

ISBN: 978-1416046967

Content Strategy Director: Mary Gatsch
Content Strategist: Michael Houston
Content Development Specialist: Rachel Miller
Publishing Services Manager: Julie Eddy
Project Manager: Kelly Milford
Design Direction: Steven Stave

Printed in United States of America

Last digit is the print number: 9   8   7   6   5   4   3   2   1

CONTRIBUTORS

Peter E. Andersen, MD
Professor, Otolaryngology, Head and Neck Surgery
Oregon Health and Science University
Portland, Oregon

Frohar Bahiraei, MD
Whidbey General Hospital
Coupeville, Washington

David Brooks, MD
Associate Professor of Surgery
Harvard Medical School
Director of Minimally Invasive Surgery
Brigham and Women's Hospital
Boston, Massachusetts

L. Michael Brunt, MD
Professor of Surgery
Department of Surgery, Institute for Minimally
   Invasive Surgery
Washington University School of Medicine
St. Louis, Missouri

Lily Chang, MD, FACS
Department of General Surgery
Virginia Mason Medical Center
Seattle, Washington

Robert Cima, MD
Associate Professor and Consultant
Department of Surgery
Mayo Clinic College of Medicine
Rochester, Minnesota

Gregory F. Dakin, MD, FACS
Associate Professor of Surgery,
Weill-Cornell Medical College
New York, New York

Daniel Davis, DO, FACS
Chief of Bariatric Surgery, Stamford Hospital
Assistant Professor of Surgery, Columbia University
Stamford, Connecticut

James Dolan, MD
Assistant Professor of Surgery, Department of Surgery
Oregon Health and Science University
Portland, Oregon

Eric Dozois, MD
Professor of Surgery, Department of Surgery
Division of Colon and Rectal Surgery, Mayo Clinic
Rochester, Minnesota

David B. Earle, MD, FACS
Director, Minimally Invasive Surgery
Baystate Medical Center
Assistant Professor of Surgery
Tufts University School of Medicine
Springfield, Massachusetts

Heidi L. Elliott, MD
Department of Minimally Invasive and General
   Surgery
Lawrence and Memorial Hospital
New London, Connecticut

Jessica Evans, MD
General/Minimally Invasive Surgeon, Department
   of General Surgery
Parker Adventist Hospital
Parker, Colorado
Sky Ridge Medical Center
Lone Tree, Colorado

Jonathan F. Finks, MD
Assistant Professor of Surgery
Director, Adult Bariatric Surgery Program
University of Michigan Health Systems
Ann Arbor, Michigan

Ani J. Fleisig, MD
Director of Surgical Oncology
Department of Surgery
Ventura County Medical Center
Ventura, California

Erin W. Gilbert, MD
Minimally Invasive Surgery Fellow
Department of General Surgery
Oregon Health & Science University
Portland, Oregon

Jennifer L. Irani, MD
Instructor in Surgery
Harvard Medical School
Associate Surgeon, Department of Surgery
Brigham and Women's Hospital
Dana Farber Cancer Institute
Gastrointestinal Cancer Center
Boston, Massachusetts

Blair Jobe, MD, FACS
Professor of Surgery
University of Pittsburgh
Pittsburgh, Pennsylvania

Daniel B. Jones, MD, MS, FACS
Vice Chair of Surgery, Office of Technology
    and Innovation
Professor in Surgery, Harvard Medical School
Chief, Minimally Invasive Surgical Services
Beth Israel Deaconess Medical Center
Boston, Massachusetts

Lauren Kosinski, MD
Assistant Professor, Department of Surgery
Section of Colon and Rectal Surgery
Medical College of Wisconsin
Milwaukee, Wisconsin

David Larson, MD, FACS
Associate Professor of Surgery
Vice Chair of Practice Department Surgery
Consultant, Department of Surgery
Division of Colon and Rectal Surgery
    Mayo Clinic
Rochester, Minnesota

David Lautz, MD
Director of Bariatric Surgery, Harvard Medical School
Department of Surgery, Brigham and Women's
    Hospital
Boston, Massachusetts

Robert Lim, MD
Clinical Fellow, Department of Minimally
    Invasive Surgery
Beth Israel Deaconess Medical Center
Boston, Massachusetts
Lieutenant Colonel, Medical Corps
United States Army

Kirk Ludwig, MD
The Vernon O. Underwood Professor
Associate Professor of Surgery
Chief, Division of Colorectal Surgery
Department of Surgery
Medical College of Wisconsin
Milwaukee, Wisconsin

Gregory J. Mancini, MD
Assistant Professor of Surgery
University of Tennessee Graduate School of Medicine
Knoxville, Tennessee

Matthew L. Mancini, MD
Associate Professor of Surgery
University of Tennessee Graduate School of Medicine
Knoxville, Tennessee

Matthew T. Menard, MD
Co-Director, Endovascular Surgery
Associate Surgeon, Division of Vascular
    and Endovascular Surgery,
Brigham and Women's Hospital
Harvard Medical School
Boston, Massachusetts

Corey Ming-Lum, MD
Minimally Invasive Surgery Fellow, Department
    of Surgery
Division of Minimally Invasive Surgery
Washington University School of Medicine
Saint Louis, Missouri

Edward C. Mun, MD
Clinical Faculty, Department of Surgery
UCLA Harbor General
Torrance, California
Staff Surgeon, Department of Surgery
Kaiser Permanente South Bay Medical Center
Harbor City, California

Nicholas O'Rourke, MBBS, FRACS
Consulting Surgeon
Royal Brisbane Hospital
Brisbane, Australia

Brant Oelschlager, MD
Byers Professor for Esophageal Research
Chief, Gastrointestinal Surgery
Director, Center for Videoendoscopic Surgery
University of Washington School of Medicine
Seattle, Washington

Emma Patterson, MD
Medical Director
Bariatric Surgery Program
Legacy Good Samaritan Medical Center
Portland, Oregon

Thai Pham, MD
Assistant Professor of Surgery,
North Texas Veteran Affairs Health Care System
University of Texas Southwestern,
Dallas, Texas

Alfons Pomp, MD
Leon C. Hirsch Professor of Surgery
Weill-Cornell Medical College
New York, New York

David Rattner, MD
Professor of Surgery
Harvard Medical School
Boston, Massachusetts

Chandrajit P. Raut, MD, MSc
Division of Surgical Oncology
Brigham and Women's Hospital
Center for Sarcoma and Bone Oncology
Dana-Farber Cancer Institute
Assistant Professor of Surgery
Harvard Medical School
Boston, Massachusetts

William P. Robinson III, MD
Assistant Professor of Surgery
Division of Vascular and Endovascular Surgery
University of Massachusetts Medical School
UMass Memorial Medical Center

Joshua S. Schindler, MD
Medical Director, OHSU-Northwest Clinic for Voice
    and Swallowing
Assistant Professor, OHSU Department
    of Otolaryngology,
Portland, Oregon

Brett C. Sheppard, MD, FACS
Professor and Clinical Vice-Chairman of Surgery
William E. Colson Chair for Pancreatic Disease
    Research
PI- Oregon Pancreas Tumor Registry
Foregut and Pancreatico-Hepatobiliary Multi-
    Disciplinary Working Groups
Division of Gastrointestinal and General Surgery
Oregon Health & Science University (OHSU)
Department of Surgery
Portland, Oregon

Douglas S. Smink, MD, MPH
Department of Surgery
Brigham and Women's Hospital
Assistant Professor of Surgery
Harvard Medical School
Boston, Massachusetts

Mark Smith, MBChB, MMed Sci, FRACS
Attending Bariatric Surgeon
Oregon Weight Loss Surgery and Legacy Good
    Samaritan Hospital
Portland, Oregon

Patricia Sylla, MD
Assistant Professor of Surgery, Harvard Medical School
Department of Surgery
Massachusetts General Hospital
Boston, Massachusetts

Ali Tavakkolizadeh, MD
Department of Surgery, Brigham and Women's
    Hospital
Assistant Professor of Surgery, Harvard Medical School
Boston, Massachusetts

Swee H. Teh, MD, FACS, FRCSI
Medical Director
Hepatibiliary Surgery
Sacred Heart Medical Center
Eugene, Oregon

Ashley H. Vernon, MD
Associate Surgeon, Division of General
    and Gastrointestinal Surgery
Brigham and Women's Hospital
Boston, Massachusetts

Mark Whiteford, MD
Director, Colon and Rectal Surgery
Providence Cancer Center
Surgeon, Gastrointestinal & Minimally Invasive
    Surgery Division
The Oregon Clinic
Affiliate Associate Professor of Surgery, Oregon Health
    & Science University
Portland, Oregon

Gordon Wisbach, MD, FACS
Director of Minimally Invasive & Bariatric Surgery,
    General Surgery Department
Naval Medical Center San Diego
San Diego, California
Assistant Professor of Surgery, F. Edward Hebert
    School of Medicine
Uniformed Services University of the Health Sciences
Bethesda, MD

Bart Witteman, MD
Research Fellow
Division of Thoracic and Foregut Surgery
University of Pittsburgh
Pittsburgh, Pennsylvania

Dedication

To all of you who are pleased that this atlas is completed! This includes not only our readers but particularly our families and colleagues at Brigham & Women's Hospital who have supported us.

—**Ashley H. Vernon, MD**

—**Stanley W. Ashley, MD**

FOREWORD

"A picture is worth a thousand words"

This atlas is for the practicing surgeon, surgical residents and medical students for their review and preparation for surgical procedures. New procedures are developed and old ones are replaced as technologic and pharmacologic advances occur. The topics presented are contemporaneous surgical procedures with step by step illustrations, along with the preoperative and postoperative considerations as well as pearls and pitfalls, taken from the personal experience and surgical practice of the authors. Their results have been validated in their surgical practices involving many patients. Operative surgery remains a manual art in which the knowledge, judgment and technical skill of the surgeon come together for the benefit of the patient. A technically perfect operation is the key to this success. Speed in operation comes from having a plan and devoting sufficient time to completion of each step, in order one time. The surgeon must be dedicated to spending the time to do it right the first time; if not, there will never be enough time to do it right at any other time. Use this atlas, study it for your patients.

"an amateur practices until he gets it right; a professional practices until she can't get it wrong"

Courtney M. Townsend, Jr., MD

B. Mark Evers, MD

PREFACE

Minimally invasive surgery continues to evolve. Although basic principles established with the introduction of laparoscopic cholecystectomy remain valid, operative approaches and technical modifications have been introduced rapidly and to considerable benefit. Although there have been several excellent laparoscopic atlases, in this context we felt that another addition to this literature was not only appropriate but needed, particularly if we could take a unique approach to the presentation.

To this end, we have tried to combine what we believe are the best aspects of previous texts. Specifically, we have included both illustrations and video in parallel. Compared with traditional open procedures which are considerably more difficult to capture and illustrate photographically, minimally invasive surgery is in fact defined by its video "nature." Despite this, we believe that illustrations can focus the emphasis in a fashion that can be lost with exclusively video images. However, to maintain video validity and permit cross-referencing, we have tried wherever possible to employ illustrations that provide the same perspective as that obtained with the laparoscope. In addition, rather than offer only our perspective on these techniques, we invited a group of authors whom we believe are among the most experienced in, and often the pioneers in the development of, these techniques. They were asked to describe these procedures for an audience that we hope will include both the surgical trainee and the practicing surgeon. Our authors have given expert advice on patient selection and demonstrated the best laparoscopic techniques. They have tried to guide the reader in choosing the best operating room configuration and the most useful equipment which are critical to making laparoscopic surgery comfortable for the surgeon and safe for the patient. They provide not only the basics but also, some "tricks" will make the job easier and better.

The opportunity to develop this atlas has been an honor and privilege and we appreciate Drs. Townsend and Evers's encouragement of our efforts. We would also like to thank the publisher, Elsevier, and in particular Rachel Miller and Judith Fletcher, for their unwavering support during the development. Their suggestions and attention to detail made it possible to overcome the innumerable problems that occur in developing such an atlas. The first author thanks all of her "laparoscopic" mentors along the way—Keith Georgeson, John Hunter, Brett Sheppard and David Brooks. The senior author thanks the first author—without her vision and persistence this volume would never have been completed.

—**Ashley H. Vernon, MD**

—**Stanley W. Ashley, MD**

TABLE OF CONTENTS

VIDEO TABLE OF CONTENTS

Access all videos online at expertconsult.com. See inside front cover for activation code.

I

Upper Gastrointestinal Surgery

ZENKER'S DIVERTICULUM

Peter E. Andersen and Joshua S. Schindler

Step 1. Surgical Anatomy

- Zenker's diverticulum is a pulsion diverticulum that occurs between the lowermost fibers of the inferior pharyngeal constrictor and the cricopharyngeal (CP) segment. This segment is the upper esophageal sphincter (UES) and is composed of the cricopharyngeus muscle and a portion of the upper esophagus musculature (Figure 1-1).
- The etiology of Zenker's diverticulum is a failure of timely opening of the CP segment. The diverticular sac forms in a relative weak spot in the posterior pharyngeal wall as contraction of the tongue and pharyngeal musculature builds pressure above a closed CP segment. Therefore, surgical correction of the condition must address not only the diverticulum but also the hypertonic or stenotic CP segment by performing a thorough myotomy.
- The transoral approach provides easy access to the diverticular sac and the CP segment (which lies within the common wall between the diverticulum and the cervical esophagus). However, the access to the segment is limited by the size of the diverticulum. Therefore, it is paradoxically easier to perform an adequate operation on patients with large diverticula as these may be stapled. Diverticula smaller than 2.5 cm may be inadequately divided by stapling because of limitations of the device and inadequate access to the CP segment. However, these smaller diverticula may be treated endoscopically with a CO_2 laser in similar fashion.
- The availability of endostapling devices has decreased the concern of postoperative salivary leakage to a minimum. Improvements in laser technology allow this laser division to be performed safely without hemorrhage or stenosis.

Step 2. Preoperative Considerations

Patient Preparation

- Patients with Zenker's diverticulum need a complete head and neck examination to identify other anatomic or neurologic causes for dysphagia. The input of a speech-language pathologist trained in dysphagia is extremely helpful. Many of these patients are elderly and may have more than one reason for their dysphagia. The symptom of dysphagia may not improve after repair of the Zenker's diverticulum if other contributing causes are not identified preoperatively; in rare cases (listed later), symptoms may actually worsen.

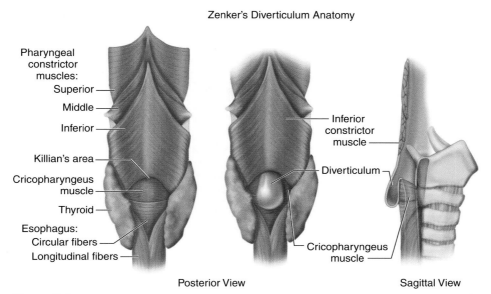

Zenker's Diverticulum Anatomy

Pharyngeal
constrictor
muscles:
    Superior
    Middle
    Inferior

Killian's area
Cricopharyngeus
muscle
Thyroid

Esophagus:
    Circular fibers
    Longitudinal fibers

Posterior View

Inferior
constrictor
muscle

Diverticulum

Cricopharyngeus
muscle

Sagittal View

Figure 1-1

Imaging

Modified barium swallow may identify pharyngeal dysphagia not seen in simple esophagram. Whichever study is performed, evaluation of bolus transit through the esophagus and lower esophageal sphincter (LES) is critical to rule out other disease processes that will not improve with surgery. When a straightforward diverticulum is seen, then the endoscopic diverticulectomy may be considered (Figure 1-2).

Pay attention to esophageal pathology distal to diverticulum. Failure to deal with these will result in a suboptimal result.

- The imaging study may identify other causes of dysphagia such as the following:
  - ▲ Diffuse esophageal spasm (Figure 1-3)
  - ▲ A distal esophageal spasm due to reflux disease
- Other findings on imaging studies must be ruled out to prevent intractable reflux following division of the UES:
  - ▲ Delayed transit (>20 seconds) through the esophagus
  - ▲ Significant reflux through a patulous LES

Body Habitus

The endoscopic repair of Zenker's diverticulum may be difficult in patients with poor mouth opening or neck extension.

Anesthesia

- General anesthetic is used with the patient orally intubated. If performing laser division, a reflective, laser-safe endotracheal tube should be used. Oxygen concentration should be maintained below 30% and diluted with helium.
- Prophylactic antibiotics that cover oral flora are given in the event that perforation of the sac occurs or there is a need to convert to open repair. We use ampicillin/sulbactam (3 gms intravenously) or clindamycin (600 mg intravenously) for the patient who is allergic to penicillins.

Positioning

- The patient is positioned supine. A shoulder roll or extension of the neck may be helpful for rigid access to the esophagus.

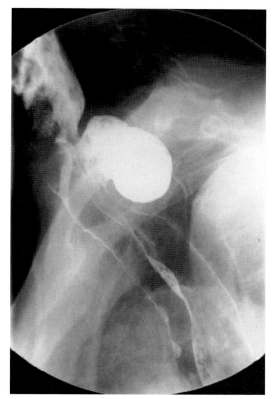

Figure 1-2

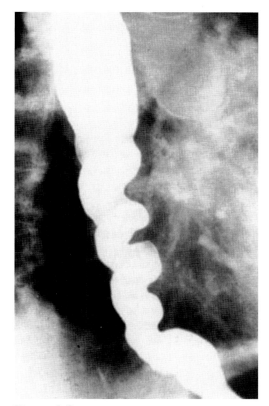

Figure 1-3

Step 3. Operative Steps

Staple-Assisted Procedure

- The Kastenbauer-Wollenberg diverticuloscope (Figure 1-4) is inserted into the mouth and passed into the hypopharynx. The anterior (longer) bill of the diverticuloscope is inserted into the introitus of the esophagus and the diverticuloscope is opened, revealing the diverticulum and the common wall between the diverticulum and the cervical esophagus. The scope is held with a suspension arm positioned on the Mayo stand (Figure 1-5).
- Because of the size of the Endo GIA 30 stapler (Covidien, Mansfield, Massachusetts), it is not possible to perform the procedure under line-of-sight vision through the diverticuloscope. Therefore, the procedure must be done using an endoscopic camera and video monitor.
- The Endo stapler is inserted into the diverticuloscope under video guidance. We prefer to place the blade that contains the refillable cartridge into the cervical esophagus (Figure 1-6).
- The Endo stapler is fired and withdrawn, revealing the divided common wall between the diverticulum and the cervical esophagus with the divided cricopharyngeus muscle (Figure 1-7).
- The diverticuloscope is removed and the patient awakened from anesthesia.

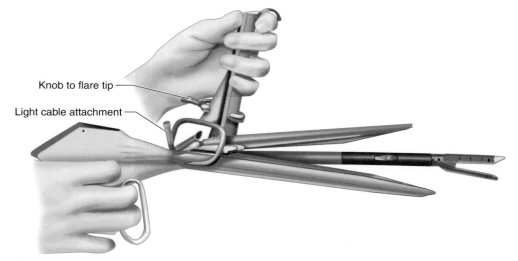

Knob to flare tip

Light cable attachment

Figure 1-4

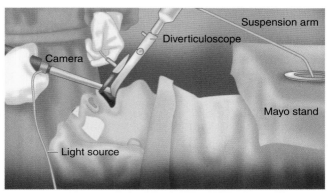

Suspension arm

Diverticuloscope

Camera

Mayo stand

Light source

Figure 1-5

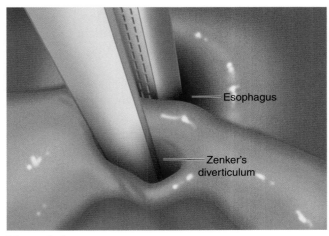

Esophagus

Zenker's diverticulum

Figure 1-6

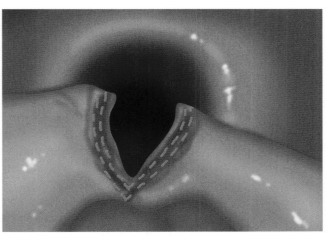

Figure 1-7

Laser-Assisted Procedure

- Positioning and exposure is performed just as with the staple-assisted procedure. The face and eyes are protected with soaking wet towels and eye shields.
- An operating microscope is used to visualize the shared wall between the diverticulum and the esophagus. The CO_2 laser is attached to a micromanipulator to direct the Helium-Neon (HeNe) aiming spot. Spot size is reduced to less than a millimeter, and the laser is used in Ultrapulse or SurgiTouch mode to maximize thermal relaxation time and minimize thermal damage. An adequate spot size (around 1 mm) will allow cutting and cauterization to proceed simultaneously.
- Incision begins through the mucosa over the superior aspect of the shared wall.
- Once opened, the transverse fibers of the cricopharyngeus may be seen. These are carefully divided to and, ultimately, through the fascia of the CP muscle at its inferior-most extent. The surgeon will know when this has been accomplished because the CP muscle will separate widely and retract into the lateral pharyngeal mucosa out of sight (Figure 1-8). A mucosal incision is made in the shared wall with a laser, showing muscle CP fibers.
- Beyond the CP muscle lies fibrous tissue posteriorly and smooth muscle of the cervical esophagus anteriorly. The upper portion of the esophageal muscle is divided as in open CP myotomy. This should not be taken to the same plane as the posterior wall of the diverticulum, but it may be taken to about 5 mm anterior to this. Posteriorly, near the anterior wall of the diverticulum, the fibrous bands should be divided to within about 5 mm of the base of the sac. Careful attention must be paid to avoid injury to the investing fascia of the pharynx and esophagus that surrounds the sac. Preservation of this fascia prevents perforation and mediastinitis (Figure 1-9).
- The mucosal incision is not closed. A 10 Fr styletted feeding tube is placed transnasally and passed into the esophagus under direct visualization. The diverticuloscope is removed carefully, the feeding tube secured to the nasal dorsum, and the patient is awakened.

Step 4. Postoperative Care

- In medically suitable patients, the staple-assisted procedure can be done on an outpatient basis. A clear liquid diet is resumed immediately and advanced as tolerated by the patient. We observe these patients for 2 to 4 hours prior to discharge to ensure that there are no problems with resuming an oral diet.
- Following laser-assisted procedures, we do prefer to observe the patient overnight. Signs of perforation and mediastinitis include fever, chest pain, malaise, and severe odynophagia. If there are no signs of a problem, an esophagram may be performed with water-soluble contrast (e.g., Gastrografin) the following morning to exclude perforation. If a small leak is noted and the patient is minimally symptomatic, the patient may be observed with nasogastric feeding for 3 to 7 days. Larger leaks and hemodynamically affected patients should be explored.
- If cleared of leak by esophagram, we remove the feeding tube and discharge on a full liquid diet. Patients may advance to a soft diet over the next 2 weeks and an unrestricted diet within a month following the procedure. We encourage clear liquids following meals to prevent stasis in the posterior pharyngeal defect.

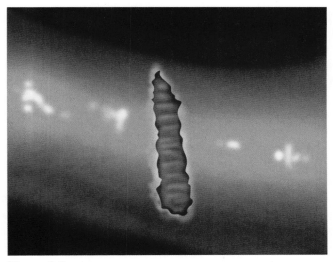

Figure 1-8

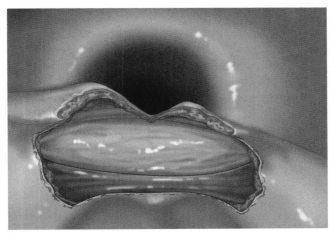

Figure 1-9

Step 5. Pearls and Pitfalls

- The endoscopic repair of Zenker's diverticula using an endostapling device is best done on patients with large sacs. We suggest that early on in a surgeon's experience only diverticula larger than 3 cm be attempted. There does not seem to be an upper limit to diverticulum size for endoscopic treatment, and the endostapler may be fired multiple times to achieve adequate marsupialization. These patients may have more esophageal dysphagia, however.
- Care must be taken to ensure that the patient does not have other esophageal pathology in addition to the Zenker's diverticulum. As this procedure will only address the dysphagia secondary to the diverticulum, failure to recognize other pathology will lead to suboptimal results. Thus, the input of an experienced speech/language pathologist and modified barium swallow rather than sole review of still images from an esophagram is prudent in the preoperative evaluation.
- Patients who cannot open their mouth widely, have large or loose upper incisor teeth, and cannot extend their neck well may be poor candidates for this approach, as the visualization of the diverticulum may be poor. It is often difficult to tell preoperatively who will be difficult to visualize. In questionable cases, the surgeon and patient may decide to proceed with traditional external approaches at the same procedure if the endoscopic approach is not feasible.
- Following the immediate healing period, postoperative esophagrams are not done unless the patient continues to be symptomatic. It is important to point out that the diverticular sac is not removed in this procedure. It is simply marsupialized into the cervical esophagus and a thorough cricopharyngeal myotomy is performed. Therefore, if a postoperative esophagram is performed, a diverticulum will still be present. For this reason the success or failure cannot be judged on radiographic studies but must be based solely on patient symptoms.

Selected References

Adams J, Sheppard B, Andersen P, et al: Zenker's diverticulostomy with cricopharyngeal myotomy: the endoscopic approach. *Surg Endosc* 15(1):34-37, 2001.
Gross N, Cohen J, Andersen P: Outpatient endoscopic Zenker diverticulectomy. *Laryngoscope* 114(2):208-11, 2004.
Lippert BM, Folz BJ, Rudert HH, et al: Management of Zenker's diverticulum and postlaryngectomy pseudodiverticulum with the CO2 laser. *Otolaryngol Head Neck Surg* 121(6):909-14, 1999.
Veenker EA, Andersen PE, Cohen JI: Cricopharyngeal spasm and Zenker's diverticulum. *Head Neck,* 25(8):681-94, 2003.

CHAPTER 2

MINIMALLY INVASIVE ESOPHAGECTOMY

Bart P.L. Witteman and Blair A. Jobe

Step 1. Surgical Anatomy

- Adenocarcinoma is the most common type of esophageal cancer in Western society, and esophagectomy is the primary therapy for resectable tumors. Traditional "open" esophagectomy has been associated with significant morbidity and mortality rates. In an attempt to lower these rates, minimally invasive techniques were introduced. Two laparoscopic approaches, each indicated for different stages of disease, are described in this chapter.
- Laparoscopic transhiatal inversion esophagectomy (LIE) with gastric substitution can be employed for treatment of end-stage benign disease (Barrett's high-grade dysplasia; achalasia) and early malignancy confined to the mucosa (T1a stage).
- Esophageal cancer is known for early and rapid dissemination because of the longitudinally oriented lymphatic plexus within the submucosa with direct transmural lymphatic connections and the lack of a serosal lining. Although lymph node involvement is infrequent in T1a-stage adenocarcinoma of the esophagus, lymph node involvement increases nearly 10-fold in T1b-stage (submucosal) disease.
- The combined laparoscopic-thoracoscopic (two-cavity) approach with en bloc lymphadenectomy is indicated for treatment of resectable advanced locoregional disease.

Step 2. Preoperative Considerations

Patient Preparation

- Preoperative evaluation and staging includes endoscopy, bronchoscopy, endosonography and positron emission tomography combined with computed tomography (PET-CT) scanning.
- Preoperative evaluation of comorbid conditions should include at least an evaluation of a patient's cardiopulmonary reserve. In selected cases with severe peripheral occlusive arterial disease, a visceral angiogram is obtained.
- A preoperative exercise program, smoking cessation, and optimization of nutritional status should be endeavored.
- Preoperative mechanical bowel preparation is performed when colon interposition may be required.

Equipment and Instrumentation

- Padded footboard
- Blunt port (Covidien, Mansfield, Massachusetts) 5 to 12 mm
- Port 5 mm (4)
- 30-degree and 45-degree 10 mm endoscope and a 5-mm 30-degree endoscope
- Needle feeding jejunostomy kit (Compat Biosystems, Minneapolis, Minnesota)
- Autosonix ultrasonic scalpel (Covidien, Mansfield, Massachusetts)
- Diamond-flex liver retractor or Nathanson liver retractor for left lobe of liver
- Endoscopic retractor (10 mm) for retracting lung
- Large endoscopic clips applier
- ½ inch Penrose drain 18 inches, cut in half

Anesthesia

- Prior to induction, a thoracic epidural is placed for postoperative pain control, and antibiotic prophylaxis (second-generation cephalosporin) is administered.
- Endotracheal intubation is performed with a single lumen tube in LIE. In combined laparoscopic-thoracoscopic (two-cavity)-approach, a double lumen endotracheal tube is required for single-lung ventilation.
- A nasogastric tube and a urinary catheter are placed, and an arterial catheter for continuous blood pressure monitoring is instituted.

Step 3. Operative Steps

Laparoscopic Transhiatal Inversion Esophagectomy

Patient Positioning

- After induction, an intraoperative bronchoscopy and esophagogastroduodenoscopy are performed for assessment of anatomic relationships and tumor location.
- Skin preparation and draping of the abdomen, chest, and left side of the neck is performed in a single field.
- For the abdominal portion of laparoscopic esophagectomy, the patient is placed in a supine, split-legged position and secured to the operation table with supportive padding for all pressure zones. A cushion can be placed at scapula level to induce slight neck extension for cervical exposure, if a neck anastomosis is planned.
- The surgeon stands between the patient's legs (French position); the first assistant is positioned at the patient's left and the second assistant at the patient's right.

Port placement

- After pneumoperitoneum is obtained by using Veress needle technique, the primary site of access is approximately 15 cm below the left costal margin, 3 cm out of the midline. A 45-degree laparoscope is introduced through a 10-mm port and, before secondary port placements, a staging laparoscopy is performed.
- A six-port approach is used with the remaining ports in the following locations: second port (12 mm, surgeon's right hand) 12 cm from the xiphoid process, 2 cm below the left costal margin; third port (5 mm, first assistant) left anterior axillary line along the costal margin; fourth port (5 mm, liver retractor) left of the xiphoid process; fifth port (12 mm, surgeon's left hand, access endoscopic stapling device) inferior to the right costal margin and immediately to the right of the falciform ligament; sixth port (5 mm, second assistant) right midabdominal position, based on internal anatomy (Figure 2-1).

Hiatal Dissection

- Using a liver retractor, the hiatal opening and the gastrohepatic omentum are exposed and divided, along with the hepatic branch of the anterior vagus trunk, using the Harmonic scalpel (Figure 2-2).
- A replaced left hepatic artery in the lesser omentum, which arises from the left gastric artery in about 30% of population, should be spared.
- The phrenoesophageal membrane is opened around the esophagus until both the crural pillars are dissected and the esophagus can be encompassed.
- In LIE indicated for benign disease or early malignancies, the vagal nerves are preserved to maintain gastric physiology.

Gastric Mobilization

- The epiphrenic fat is retracted toward the left anterior abdominal wall to provide tension on the left gastric vessels. The overlying peritoneum is opened, using the Harmonic scalpel, and the left gastric vessels are identified and divided using an endoscopic vascular stapler (Figure 2-3).
- The gastric fundus is mobilized with the division of the short vessels.
- The gastrocolic omentum is divided along the greater curvature. At Demel's (watershed) point, the union of left and right gastroepiploic vessels is preserved to protect the blood supply to the gastric conduit (Figure 2-4).

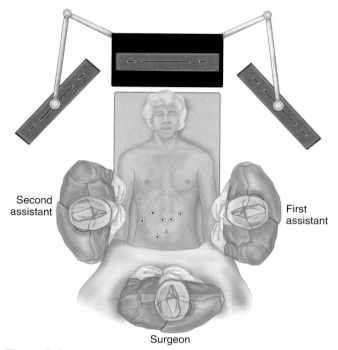

Second assistant

First assistant

Surgeon

Figure 2-1

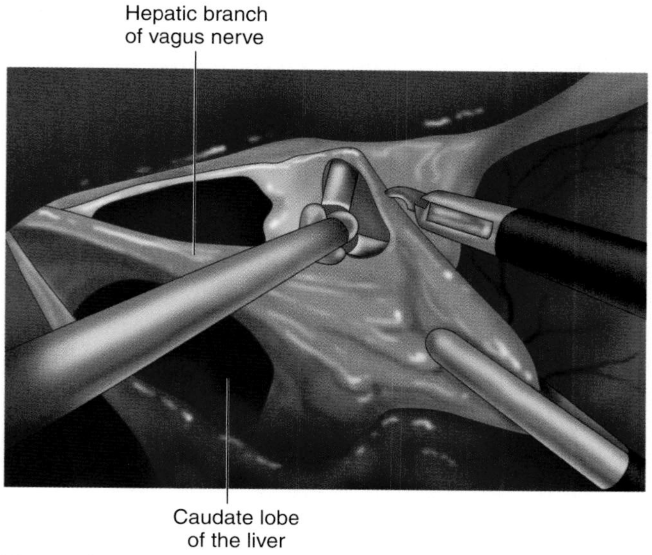

Hepatic branch of vagus nerve

Caudate lobe of the liver

Figure 2-2

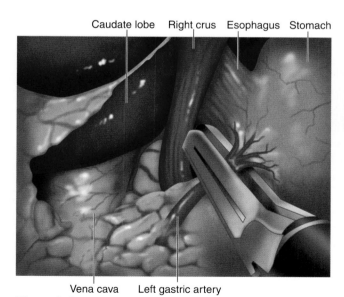

Caudate lobe   Right crus   Esophagus   Stomach

Vena cava   Left gastric artery

Figure 2-3

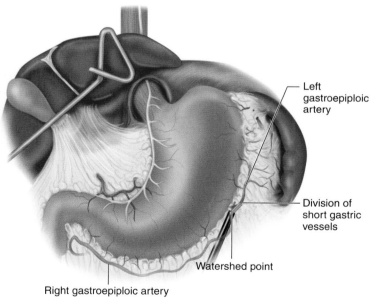

Left gastroepiploic artery

Division of short gastric vessels

Watershed point

Right gastroepiploic artery

Figure 2-4

- The gastrosplenic ligament is divided, including the intervening short gastric vessels, and the gastric fundus is further mobilized along the pancreaticogastric fold, where the posterior gastric artery is identified and divided.
- The distal stomach is mobilized by the division of the gastrocolic ligament at the greater curvature and then the attachments between the posterior gastric wall and pancreas. When the gastric duodenal artery is identified, Kocher's maneuver is performed. The duodenum and pancreas head are detached from retroperitoneum and retracted to the patient's left side. Care is taken to protect the gastroduodenal artery, to maintain blood flow to the right gastroepiploic artery to supply the gastric conduit.

Gastric Conduit Creation

- The nasogastric tube is retracted to an intrathoracic position.
- The gastric conduit is created using an endostapler (45 mm). The first load is fired 5 to 6 cm proximal to the pylorus and, stepwise, the conduit is created 5 cm from the lesser curvature. Care is taken to preserve the right gastric vessels (Figure 2-5).
- The distal margin of the lesser curvature, which is maintained in continuity with the esophagus, is resected and sent for frozen section examination intraoperatively to confirm clear resection margin.
- At this point, a pyloroplasty can be performed to prevent gastric outlet obstruction in the case of vagotomy in en bloc lymph node dissection.

Transhiatal Mobilization and Esophagogastric Division

- The distal esophagus is mobilized circumferentially in the mediastinum through the hiatus. The right crus can be divided to improve exposure. The dissection of the mediastinal portion of the esophagus from the surrounding intrathoracic structures is performed as proximally as is safe. Care is taken to prevent damage to the trachea, inferior pulmonary veins, azygos vein, and aortic arch.
- To determine the location of the anatomic esophagogastric junction, an intraoperative endoscopy is performed. The gastric fundus is divided with an endoscopic stapler, distal to the esophagogastric junction, placed in an Endobag and removed at the end of the procedure (Figure 2-6).
- A needle jejunostomy is placed for postoperative nutrition.
- In advanced disease stage, the greater curve side of the conduit tip is secured to the staple line in the distal esophagus to facilitate the gastric pull-up and the procedure is converted to a right-sided thoracoscopy for the laparoscopic-thoracoscopic (two-cavity) approach.

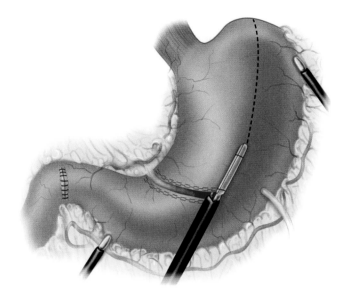

Figure 2-5

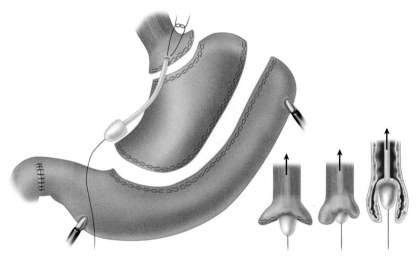

Figure 2-6

Cervical Access

◆ Access to the cervical esophagus is obtained through a 5-cm incision along the medial border of the sternocleidomastoid muscle. The platysma and omohyoid muscles are divided. Through the avascular plane, the carotid sheath is exposed and retracted laterally. The thyroid gland and the trachea are retracted medially, while attention is paid to preserve the recurrent laryngeal nerve. The deep cervical fascia is opened, and blunt fingertip dissection is used to surround the esophagus with fascia and access the upper mediastinum.

Inversion Technique

◆ The cervical esophagus is opened and a vein stripper is introduced retrograde into the esophagus. Through a small gastrotomy at staple-line level, the vein stripper is retrieved and taken out of the abdomen through the right upper abdominal 12-mm port site. A medium-sized anvil and a 60-cm trailing suture are placed on the end of the vein stripper.
◆ After retraction into the abdominal cavity, the anvil is secured with a horizontal mattress suture to the gastrotomy and the esophagus is inverted by drawing back the cervical end of the vein stripper.
◆ The inverted border of the esophagus is grasped and gentle traction at the cervical end of the vein stripper provides counter-tension to facilitate mobilization during division of mediastinal attachments and blood vessels.
◆ The dissection is continued until the esophagus is extracted through the cervical wound and transected at the proximal margin.

Conduit Pull-through and Esophagogastrostomy

◆ The 60-cm trailing suture, which was fixed at the anvil site of the vein stripper and pulled through the cervical wound with the specimen, is used to bring a 26 French thoracic drainage tube down into the abdominal cavity from the cervical incision. The proximal gastric conduit is sutured to the tube, carefully pulled through the mediastinum, and brought to the surface in the cervical wound without rotation.
◆ A vertical gastrotomy is made in the gastric conduit to allow a 3.5-mm Endo GIA stapler (Covidien, Mansfield, Massachusetts) to be inserted in the conduit and the proximal esophagus to create a stapled end-to-side anastomosis. The gastrostomy and enterotomy are closed in two layers (Figure 2-7).

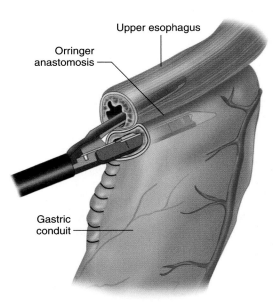

Figure 2-7

Closing

- A nasogastric tube is introduced into the gastric conduit.
- In the cervical opening, a closed suction drain is placed alongside the anastomosis, and the fascia layers and platysma muscle are closed.
- Final inspection of the abdominal cavity is performed, and the specimen retrieval bag containing the gastric fundus and all trocars are removed under direct visualization. The fascia is closed using Vicryl sutures and the skin is closed using resorbable sutures.

Combined Laparoscopic-Thoracoscopic (Two-Cavity) Approach

Positioning

- In this approach, the patient is intubated with a double-lumen tube for single-lung ventilation during the thoracic part of the procedure.
- The abdominal portion of the procedure is carried out similar to that described above for the LIE, but the inversion technique is not performed; instead, lymphatic tissue and vagal nerve branches are resected en bloc with the esophagus and esophagogastric junction.
- For thoracoscopic mobilization of the esophagus (after the abdominal portion of the procedure), the patient is repositioned into a left lateral decubitus position and supported with a beanbag. The right hemithorax is disinfected, drapes are placed, and single (right) lung ventilation is applied. The surgeon stands on the patient's right, the first assistant stands on the patient's left.

Port Placement

- Five ports are introduced: a 10-mm camera port in the 7th-8th intercostal space, midaxillary line; a 5-mm port in the 8th-9th intercostal space, posterior axillary line; a 10-mm port in the 4th intercostal space on the anterior axillary line; and a 5-mm port posterior to the scapula tip (Figure 2-8). A single 5-mm port is placed anteriorly for suction.
- A staging thoracoscopy and laparoscopy is performed to evaluate the presence of gastric extension, liver metastases, peritoneal carcinomatosis, or T4 tumor.

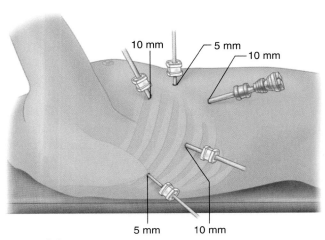

Figure 2-8

Esophageal Mobilization

- The central tendon of the diaphragm is retracted inferior-anteriorly using a percutaneous suture.
- The inferior pulmonary ligament is divided to the level of the inferior pulmonary vein and artery, and the esophagus with attached lymphatic tissues is dissected away from the pericardium and developed toward both cranial and caudal sides.
- The mediastinal pleura are opened until the azygos arch can be identified and divided using a reticulating endoscopic vascular stapling device.
- Proximal to the azygos vein, dissection must be in close proximity to the esophagus to avoid recurrent laryngeal nerve injury. The subcarinal space is developed, and the esophagus is dissected away from the right and left mainstem bronchi (Figure 2-9).
- Division of the aortoesophageal vessels is performed with special attention to the preservation of the contralateral pleura and the thoracic duct.

Conduit Pull-through and Esophagogastrostomy

- The esophagus is mobilized into the abdominal-thoracic inlet and separated from the hiatus.
- The conduit that is attached via a suture to the specimen is pulled intramediastinally through the hiatus. The suture is cut and the specimen is retracted in a cranial direction, thereby exposing the most medial aspect of the mediastinal dissection (e.g., contralateral pleura).
- The upper esophagus is divided 3 cm cranially to the azygos vein level using endoscopic scissors, and the specimen is removed through the extended surgeon right-hand port using a wound protector. The specimen is opened and checked for gross margins.

Intrathoracic Anastomosis

- The esophageal-conduit anastomosis is created using a 28 mm endoscopic end-to-end stapler (Ivor-Lewis approach). The anvil is sutured into the proximal esophagus, and the conduit staple line is opened to allow access of a stapler that is introduced intrathoracically through the extended inferior posterolateral port (Figure 2-9).
- Rotation must be prevented and the length of conduit necessary to achieve a tensionless anastomosis must be determined. The presence of tissue "doughnuts" in the stapler after firing is confirmed, as this indicates a complete circumferential anastomosis. Closure of the gastrotomy is performed by dividing the surplus conduit with a roticulating endoscopic stapler and removed. This specimen will serve as the final distal margin for histologic examination.
- A nasogastric tube is placed in the conduit proximal to the hiatal opening and a Jackson-Pratt drain is placed near the anastomosis opposite from the staple line. After the thoracic cavity is irrigated with warmed antibiotic saline, hemostasis is achieved and the right lung is re-ventilated after placement of a 28 French thoracostomy tube.

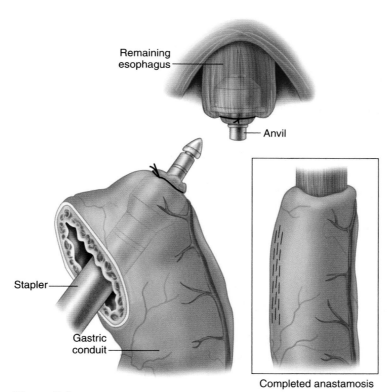

Figure 2-9

Closing

♦ The fascia is closed using Vicryl suture, and skin is closed with resorbable suture.
♦ The double-lumen tube is exchanged for a single-lumen tube, and a bronchoscopy is performed to clear intrapulmonary secretions.

Step 4. Postoperative Care

General rules for postoperative care after minimally invasive esophagectomy:
♦ Early ambulation and pulmonary physiotherapy are initiated.
♦ The nasogastric tube is removed and jejunostomy tube feeding is started around the third postoperative day if there is no sign of ileus.
♦ Dietary education is provided and is focused on small, frequent meals.
♦ Before discharge, an upper GI-tract contrast x-ray is performed (on the 6th to 7th postoperative day) to verify the integrity of the anastomosis and pyloroplasty.
♦ An evaluation visit is scheduled at 2 to 3 weeks, and the jejunostomy is removed at 6 weeks if the patient's oral intake and weight are sufficient.
♦ The closed suction drain is pulled back by 2 cm prior to discharge. This drain is removed at the first postoperative clinic visit after the patient undergoes an upper gastrointestinal contrast radiographic examination.

Step 5. Pearls and Pitfalls

♦ In addition to the techniques described in this chapter, other successful minimally invasive approaches have been reported. The key to success for minimally invasive esophagectomy is a high patient volume and a well-trained multidisciplinary surgical team.
♦ Neoadjuvant chemotherapy is not seen as a contraindication to the minimally invasive approach.
♦ LIE can be used for lesions across the esophagogastric junction by the use of an antegrade (proximal to distal) inversion technique. The inversion starts in the proximal esophagus and the esophagus is extracted through an abdominal port site.
♦ If vagotomy is performed, a gastric drainage procedure (pyloroplasty, pyloromyotomy, or pyloric finger disruption) is performed, at the surgeon's discretion, to prevent delayed gastric emptying and associated complications (e.g., aspiration pneumonia). We routinely perform pyloroplasty following a vagotomy; however, this procedure is controversial because it could induce bile reflux into the conduit and contribute to anastomotic stricture development.
  ▲ Pyloriplasty—Heineke and Mikulicz technique: superior and inferior tension sutures are placed. The muscular layer is incised using ultrasonic scissors and subsequently closed transversally with interrupted sutures (Figure 2-10).

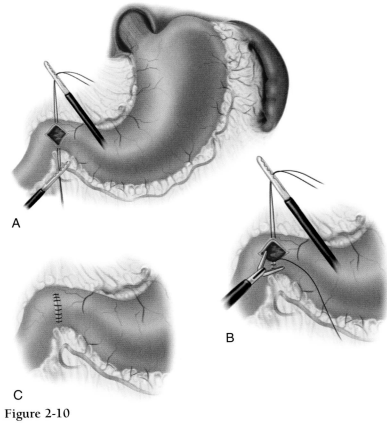

A

B

C

Figure 2-10

- ◆ The Ivor-Lewis approach in the combined laparoscopic-thoracoscopic (two-cavity) esophagectomy with thoracoscopic intrathoracic anastomosis can be employed only for lesions in the distal third of the esophagus. For more proximal lesions, a cervical anastomosis is advised.

Selected References

Akiyama H, Tsurumaru M, Ono Y, et al: Esophagectomy without thoracotomy with vagal preservation. *J Am Coll Surg* 178(1):83-85, 1994.

Banki F, Mason RJ, DeMeester SR, et al: Vagal-sparing esophagectomy: a more physiologic alternative. *Ann Surg* 236(3):324-35; discussion 335-36, 2002.

Luketich JD, Alvelo-Rivera M, Buenaventura PO, et al: Minimally invasive esophagectomy: outcomes in 222 patients. *Ann Surg* 238(4):486-94; discussion 494-95, 2003.

Luketich JD, Nguyen NT, Weigel T, et al: Minimally invasive approach to esophagectomy. *JSLS* 2(3):243-47, 1998.

Jobe BA, Kim CY, Minjarez RC, et al: Simplifying minimally invasive transhiatal esophagectomy with the inversion approach: lessons learned from the first 20 cases. *Arch Surg* 141(9):857-65; discussion 865-66, 2006.

Orringer MB, Marshall B, Iannettoni MD: Eliminating the cervical esophagogastric anastomotic leak with a side-to-side stapled anastomosis. *J Thorac Cardiovasc Surg* 119(2):277-88, 2000.

Swanstrom LL, Hansen P: Laparoscopic total esophagectomy. *Arch Surg* 132(9):943-47; discussion 947-9, 1997.

CHAPTER 3

HELLER MYOTOMY WITH TOUPET OR DOR FUNDOPLICATION FOR ACHALASIA

Ani J. Fleisig and Brant K. Oelschlager

Step 1. Clinical Anatomy

- The sling fibers of Willis on the cardia of the stomach provide some competency of the lower esophageal sphincter (LES). Therefore, to completely obliterate these fibers, the myotomy should be carried at least 3 cm onto the stomach.
- To ensure an adequate myotomy onto the stomach, both the cardioesophageal fat pad and anterior (left) vagus should be mobilized as they cover the portion of cardia that is included in the myotomy.
- In patients with end-stage achalasia and a dilated sigmoid esophagus, the gastroesophageal (GE) junction is often angulated. Therefore, consideration for not doing a fundoplication should be given lest the distal esophagus be angulated more.

Step 2. Preoperative Considerations

- Manometry is essential to make the diagnosis, demonstrating an aperistaltic esophagus and an incomplete relaxation of the LES.
- Upper endoscopy and fluoroscopic evaluation should be used to exclude other pathology and to determine the amount of esophageal dilation.
- In patients over 50 years of age, symptoms less than 6 months, or those with significant weight loss (>10 to 20 lbs), CT scan or endoscopic ultrasound should be performed to rule out pseudoachalasia (i.e., a tumor obstructing the esophagus).
- In patients with atypical presentations, botulinum toxin A (Botox) can be used as a diagnostic tool to identify those who would benefit from a myotomy.

Positioning

- Patients are placed in modified lithotomy with both arms tucked.
- A beanbag overhangs the edge of the operative table to form a saddle around the patient's perineum to avoid sliding.
- The operative surgeon stands between the patient's legs with the assistant at the patient's left side.
- Monitors are placed above the patient's head.
- An oral-gastric tube can be used to decompress the stomach and then removed.
- After port placement, the patient is placed in steep reverse Trendelenburg position.

Step 3. Operative Steps

Port Placement

- A small incision is made at the left costal margin in the mid-clavicular line.
- Pneumoperitoneum is established using a Veress needle, and the abdomen is entered using a Visiport trocar (Covidien; Mansfield, Massachusetts).
- The camera port is placed 4 cm left of midline and one hand's breadth (approximately 10-12 cm) inferior to the left costal margin.
- A 10-mm 30-degree laparoscope camera provides superior visualization.
- The remaining four ports are placed under direct visualization.
- A 5-mm trocar is placed in the right upper quadrant (surgeon's left hand), a 10-mm trocar is placed in the right lateral quadrant (paddle liver retractor), and 10-mm trocar is placed in the left lower quadrant (assistant port) (Figure 3-1).

Mobilization of Esophagus

- The left phrenogastric ligament is divided to expose the left crus.
- The gastric fundus is mobilized by dividing the short gastric vessels using an ultrasonic dissector.
- Posterior attachments between the proximal stomach and retroperitoneum are divided to minimize tension on the subsequent fundoplication.
- The left phrenoesophageal membrane is divided.
- The gastrohepatic ligament is divided and carried toward the esophageal hiatus to expose the right crus.
- The nerves of Latarjet and aberrant or accessory vessels are preserved.
- The anterior phrenoesophageal membrane is divided.
- The anterior (left) vagus is identified, protected, and separated from the esophagus.

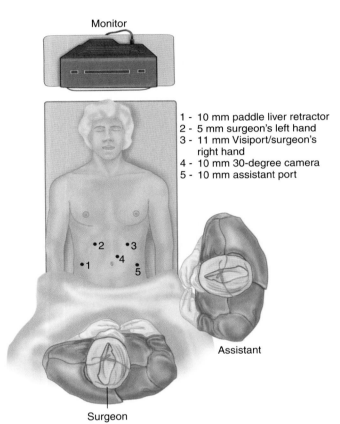

Monitor

1 - 10 mm paddle liver retractor
2 - 5 mm surgeon's left hand
3 - 11 mm Visiport/surgeon's
    right hand
4 - 10 mm 30-degree camera
5 - 10 mm assistant port

Assistant

Surgeon

Figure 3-1

- A posterior esophageal window is created, which exposes the confluence of the right and left crus.
- The posterior (right) vagus is visualized and protected.
- A Penrose drain can be placed around the GE junction to retract the esophagus during the mobilization.
- An extensive hiatal and mediastinal esophageal dissection is performed to maximize the length of the myotomy.
- The cardioesophageal fat pad attachments to the underlying stomach and esophagus are divided. In doing so, the anterior (left) vagus is preserved and separated from the GE junction.
- This fat pad to the left of the anterior (left) vagus is then resected.

Myotomy

- A lighted 50 F bougie is passed into the body of the stomach.
- A Babcock retractor is draped over the bougie, just distal to the GE junction, gently stretching the muscle fibers.
- The myotomy is performed with an L-shaped hook electrocautery device, starting on the anterior surface at the 10 o'clock position. Individual muscle fibers divide easily under gentle traction, rarely utilizing cautery.
- The longitudinal muscle fibers are divided first, exposing the inner circular muscle of the esophagus (sling fibers of Willis on the cardia). Submucosal bleeding should be controlled with pressure, not cautery (Figure 3-2).
- The myotomy should be extended as proximal as possible (6 to 8 cm) and at least 3 cm onto the cardia of the stomach.
- The bougie is removed.

Toupet Fundoplication

- The posterior gastric fundus is brought around the esophagus and secured to the right crus and to the right edge of the myotomy.
- The posterior fundus is further secured to the right by suturing it to the base of the right crus.
- A row of two or three sutures is used to attach the posterior fundus to the right side of the esophagus near the myotomy.
- In a similar fashion the anterior fundus is secured to the left crus and left edge of the myotomy.
- The hiatus is not closed, unless a large hernia is encountered.
- Upper endoscopy is performed to exclude mucosal injury during the myotomy and to ensure no resistance or angulation of the fundoplication (Figure 3-3).

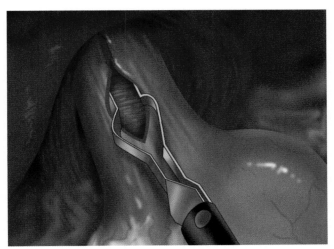

Figure 3-2

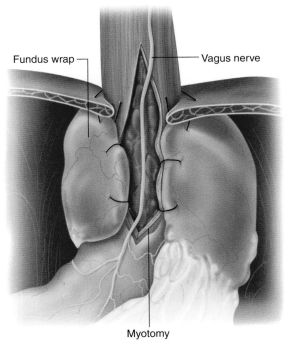

Fundus wrap

Vagus nerve

Myotomy

Figure 3-3

Dor Fundoplication

- This fundoplication folds the anterior fundus over the anterior esophagus to form an anterior flap and to re-create the angle of His. Two vertical rows of sutures are placed, one to the left (performed first) and one to the right side of the esophagus.
- The uppermost stitch incorporates the anterior gastric fundus to the left crus and left edge of the myotomy.
- The remaining two sutures are used to attach the anterior fundus to the left side of the esophagus near the myotomy, thus completing the first vertical row (Figure 3-4a).
- The gastric fundus is then folded over the esophagus from left to right to cover the myotomy.
- The greater curve of the fundus is secured to the right crus and to the right edge of the myotomy (Figure 3-4b).
- In a similar fashion, the remaining two sutures secure the fundus to the right side of the esophagus near the myotomy.
- One or two final sutures are used to secure the fundus to the anterior hiatus to prevent the fundus from angulating the esophagus at the GE junction (Figure 3-4c).
- Upper endoscopy is performed to exclude mucosal injury during the myotomy and to ensure no resistance or angulation of the fundoplication.

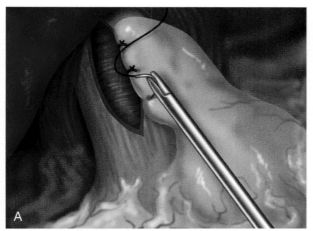

Figure 3-4a

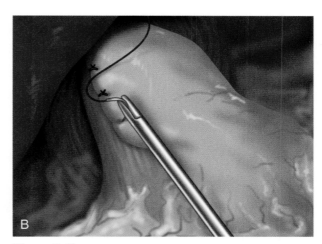

Figure 3-4b

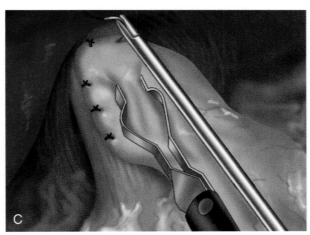

Figure 3-4c

Closure

- The paddle liver retractor should be removed under direct visualization to avoid injury to the myotomy.
- All ports are removed under direct visualization, and pneumoperitoneum is released.
- Skin and fascia are closed in the usual fashion.

Step 4. Postoperative Care

- Patients generally start liquids the night of their procedure.
- Nausea is aggressively treated with antiemetics.
- Average length of stay is 1 to 2 days.
- All medications are in liquid form for 3 to 4 weeks.
- Patients are slowly progressed from liquids to solid foods.
- Resumption of normal diet and activities occurs within 3 to 4 weeks.
- Manometry and 24-hour pH studies are performed 6 months after surgery to rule out asymptomatic but pathologic gastroesophageal reflux disease, which is present in 15% to 20% of patients.

Step 5. Pearls and Pitfalls

- The lighted bougie serves to illuminate the esophagus, shows the muscle layers to be divided, and provides a stable platform on which to perform the myotomy.
- Minimal cautery use during the myotomy prevents delayed perforations resulting from thermal mucosal injury.
- Intraoperative mucosal perforations can be repaired primarily with fine (4-0 or 5-0) absorbable suture with little or no morbidity.
- If a mucosal laceration should occur, perform a Dor fundoplication, which serves to buttress the repaired mucosa, minimizing subsequent leaks or fistulas.
- There are no data to substantiate the superiority of either Toupet or Dor fundoplication in combination with a Heller myotomy for achalasia. They each have their purported benefits. The Toupet is thought to be a better antireflux procedure and may keep the myotomy tented open. The Dor does not require taking down the short gastric vessels and can buttress the mucosa as described here.

Selected References

Richards WO, Torquati A, Holzman MD, et al: Heller myotomy versus Heller myotomy with Dor fundoplication for achalasia: a prospective randomized double-blind clinical trial. *Ann Surg* 240(3):405-12, 2004.

Woltman TA, Oelschlager BK, Pellegrini CA: Achalasia. *Surg Clin North Am* 85(3):483-93, 2005.

Wright AS, Williams CW, Pellegrini CA, et al: Long-term outcomes confirm the superior efficacy of extended Heller myotomy with Toupet fundoplication for achalasia. *Surg Endosc* 21(5):713-18, 2007.

4

NISSEN FUNDOPLICATION

Jonathan F. Finks

Step 1. Surgical Anatomy

The Antireflux Barrier

- The antireflux barrier of the gastroesophageal (GE) junction depends on proper anatomic alignment of the distal esophagus, proximal stomach, and the diaphragm. The intrinsic muscle fibers of the distal esophagus coordinate with the sling fibers of the cardia and muscle fibers of the diaphragm to prevent reflux of gastric acid into the distal esophagus (Figure 4-1).
- Tonic contraction of the sling and claps fibers of the GE junction works to maintain the acute angle of His. This contributes to the gastroesophageal flap valve mechanism, which further prevents gastroesophageal reflux (GERD) (Figure 4-2).
- Restoration of the normal anatomic position of the GE junction and re-creation of the flap valve mechanism through fundoplication are critical elements for a successful antireflux procedure.

Step 2. Preoperative Considerations

Patient Preparation

- In patients with objective evidence of gastroesophageal reflux, the indications for surgery include the following:
  - ▲ Intolerance of medical therapy or the desire to avoid lifelong medication use
  - ▲ Persistent or breakthrough symptoms despite the use of maximal medical therapy (this typically includes patients with volume reflux, or regurgitation)
  - ▲ Complications of reflux disease, including Barrett's esophagus, refractory esophagitis, and esophageal strictures
  - ▲ Supralaryngeal symptoms of reflux disease, including chronic cough, aspiration, asthma, or hoarseness

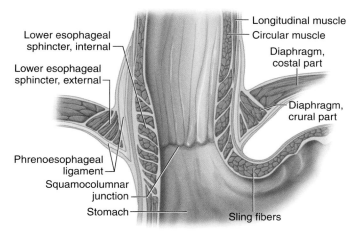

Figure 4-1

Longitudinal muscle
Circular muscle
Diaphragm, costal part
Lower esophageal sphincter, internal
Lower esophageal sphincter, external
Diaphragm, crural part
Phrenoesophageal ligament
Squamocolumnar junction
Stomach
Sling fibers

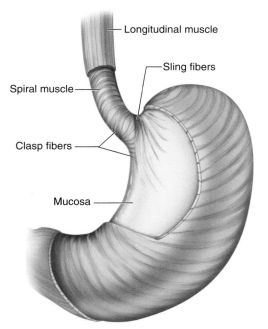

Figure 4-2

Longitudinal muscle
Sling fibers
Spiral muscle
Clasp fibers
Mucosa

- Diagnostic evaluation
  - ▲ Prior to surgical intervention, all patients require *upper endoscopy*. This provides an opportunity to evaluate the extent of esophagitis and rule out Barrett's esophagus and gastroesophageal malignancy.
  - ▲ *Esophageal manometry* is an essential study prior to antireflux surgery to rule out the presence of a severe motility disorder, such as achalasia. This is an important issue, because many of the symptoms of achalasia (regurgitation, heartburn) can mimic those of GERD, whereas the treatment is obviously very different.
  - ▲ *Ambulatory 24-hour esophageal pH* studies should be used selectively. Patients with classic reflux symptoms (heartburn and regurgitation) and esophagitis on endoscopy do not require any further evidence of GERD. However, patients with nonerosive disease and those with primarily supralaryngeal symptoms should undergo a 24-hour pH study to document the presence of abnormal reflux.
  - ▲ *Upper gastrointestinal fluoroscopic imaging* is useful for defining gastroesophageal anatomy in patients who present with dysphagia or who have previously diagnosed large hiatal hernias.
  - ▲ *A gastric emptying* study should be considered in patients presenting with significant nausea and vomiting, as these symptoms may suggest of gastroparesis, not GERD.
  - ▲ Patients with classic symptoms (heartburn and regurgitation), a good response to proton pump inhibitor therapy, and an abnormal 24-hour esophageal pH study are the most likely to benefit from antireflux surgery.

Equipment and Instrumentation

- We perform the procedure using five ports—three 5-mm ports and two 10-mm ports—as well as a 10-mm, 30-degree angled laparoscope.
- A Nathanson retractor is used to elevate the left lateral segment of the liver.
- Handheld laparoscopic instruments include atraumatic bowel graspers, scissors, and needle drivers.
- We prefer the 5-mm ultrasonic dissector for dissection and hemostasis.
- A ¼-inch, 5-cm long Penrose drain is used to facilitate retraction of the esophagus. The ends of the Penrose drain are anchored together anterior to the esophagus using a 0 chromic or Vicryl Endoloop (Covidien, Mansfield, Massachusetts).
- Permanent suture (0 silk or Ethibond, Ethicon, Somerville, New Jersey) with felt pledgets is used to close the crural defect. The fundoplication is performed with the same suture but without pledgets.
- For large crural defects (>4 cm), we use synthetic or biologic mesh to buttress the crural closure.

Anesthesia

- Prophylaxis against venous thromboembolism includes the use of sequential lower extremity compression devices and subcutaneous low molecular weight heparin.
- Perioperative antibiotics, typically a first-generation cephalosporin, are recommended.
- Following induction of general anesthesia, an orogastric tube and Foley catheter are inserted. They can be removed at the conclusion of the procedure.

Room Setup and Patient Positioning

- The patient is positioned supine with the thighs abducted. A split-leg table is preferable, although some surgeons elect to use stirrups.

Step 3. Operative Steps

Access and Port Placement

- Pneumoperitoneum is established with a Veress needle at the umbilicus or below the left costal margin.
- A 10-mm camera port is placed to the left of midline and 15 cm below the junction of the right and left costal margins. A 5-mm port is placed in the subxiphoid position. This port is then removed and replaced with the Nathanson liver retractor, which is used to elevate the left lateral segment of the liver to expose the proximal stomach and esophageal hiatus. A 10-mm port in the left upper quadrant and a 5-mm port in the right upper quadrant serve as the surgeon's two working ports, and a 5-mm assistant's port is placed laterally in the left upper quadrant (Figure 4-3).
- Following port placement, the operating table is placed into the reverse Trendelenburg position. The surgeon operates from between the legs, while the assistant stands on the patient's left side. Monitors are placed at the head of the table at eye level.
- Use of an angled 30-degree laparoscope facilitates the dissection.

Hiatal Dissection

- When present, a hiatal hernia should be reduced prior to starting the dissection in order to reduce the risk of injury to lesser curvature vessels.
- Dissection begins by opening the gastrohepatic ligament through its *pars flaccida* portion, using an ultrasonic dissector. The lesser omentum is incised superiorly to expose the right crus of the diaphragm.
- The hepatic branch of the vagus nerve, which runs through the gastrohepatic omentum, is preserved whenever possible to reduce the risk for gallstone formation.
- Up to 12% of patients will have an accessory or replaced left hepatic artery that accompanies the hepatic branch of the vagus nerve within the lesser omentum. Injury to this vessel should be avoided. If necessary for exposure, however, the vessel should be divided between hemoclips.
- The phrenoesophageal ligament anterior to the esophagus is divided with the ultrasonic dissector or hook electrocautery. It is important to open only the superficial peritoneal layers in order to avoid injury to the underlying esophagus and anterior vagus nerve (Figure 4-4).

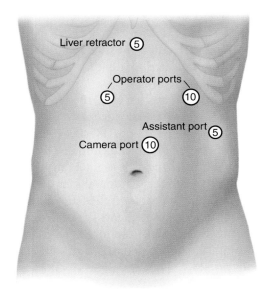

Liver retractor ⑤

Operator ports

⑤   ⑩

Assistant port ⑤

Camera port ⑩

Figure 4-3

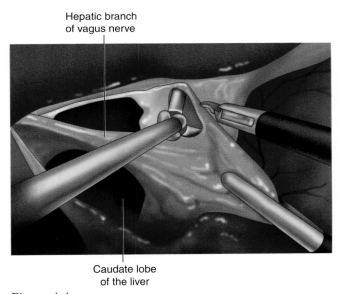

Hepatic branch
of vagus nerve

Caudate lobe
of the liver

Figure 4-4

- Retraction of the stomach to the patient's right side will facilitate exposure of the left crus. Clearance of the left crus is accomplished by dividing the peritoneal attachments between the cardia and diaphragm at the angle of His.
- With the stomach retracted to the patient's left side, the retroesophageal dissection is begun. The peritoneum anterior to the right crus is divided, and blunt dissection is used to develop a plane between the esophagus and the right crus (Figure 4-4). This dissection proceeds inferiorly toward the decussation of the right and left crura.
- Blunt dissection continues posterior to the esophagus to develop the retroesophageal window. The left crus is then identified through the window under the right side of the stomach. Blunt dissection is used to divide attachments between the left crus and the cardia of the stomach.
- The posterior vagus nerve must be identified and kept up with the esophagus during this dissection. Unlike the anterior vagus, the posterior vagus nerve often separates from the esophagus as it passes through the hiatus, making it susceptible to injury during the retroesophageal dissection.

Mobilization of the Gastric Fundus

- Complete mobilization of the fundus reduces torque on the fundoplication and may decrease the risk of postoperative dysphagia.
- Mobilization of the fundus is accomplished through division of the short gastric vessels. These are divided using the ultrasonic dissector, beginning at the level of the inferior pole of the spleen and ending at the left crus (Figure 4-5).
- The assistant facilitates exposure of the short gastric vessels initially by retracting the omentum to the patient's left, while the surgeon retracts the stomach down and to the right. However, exposure of the proximal short gastric vessels is best achieved by having the assistant retract the posterior aspect of the greater curvature toward the right side.
- Once the short gastric vessels have been divided, the remainder of the retroesophageal dissection is completed from the left side. A Penrose drain is then placed behind the esophagus and its two ends are secured anteriorly with clips or a looped suture. The Penrose drain facilitates esophageal retraction during the subsequent mediastinal dissection and crural closure.

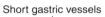
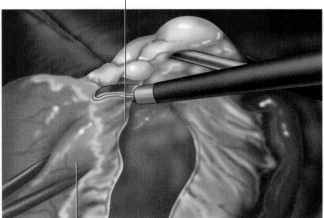

Short gastric vessels

Greater curvature

Figure 4-5

Mediastinal Dissection

- The aim of the mediastinal dissection is to mobilize the esophagus circumferentially until at least 2.5 cm to 3 cm of distal esophagus remains within the abdomen without having to apply any traction on the Penrose drain.
- This task is accomplished primarily through blunt dissection and is facilitated by dynamic retraction on the Penrose drain by the assistant. Larger feeding vessels to the esophagus should be divided with the ultrasonic dissector, but care must be taken to avoid injury to the esophagus. Mediastinal bleeding is usually easily controlled by compression with a gauze sponge inserted through a 10-mm port.
- The anterior and posterior vagus nerves should be identified and preserved from injury throughout this dissection.

Crural Closure

- The crural defect is closed using interrupted, nonabsorbable sutures and using either an intracorporeal or extracorporeal knot-tying technique (Figure 4-6).
- We use small pledgets on either side of the closure to prevent tearing through the muscle. Pledgets must be seated along the lateral aspect of the crura to prevent contact with the esophagus, as there is a risk for erosion.
- The crura should be closed loosely around the esophagus so as to avoid dysphagia.

Fundoplication

- The fundus of the stomach is pulled behind the esophagus. A "shoeshine maneuver" is performed by sliding the fundus back and forth behind the esophagus, and this ensures that the fundus has been adequately mobilized. When properly positioned, the stumps of the short gastric vessels on the fundus should line up to the right of the esophagus (Figure 4-7).

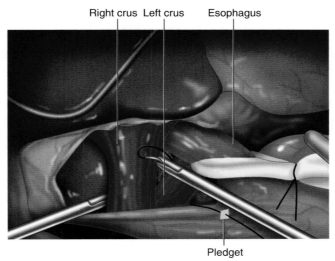

Figure 4-6

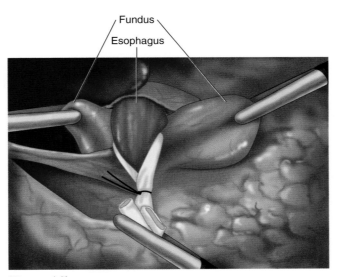

Figure 4-7

- The fundoplication is performed over a 56 French to 60 French esophageal dilator in order to ensure a "floppy" wrap, which helps minimize the risk for dysphagia. Once complete, the surgeon should be able to pass a grasper between the wrap and the esophagus easily.
- The fundoplication is accomplished using three interrupted nonabsorbable sutures. Each suture incorporates stomach on either side of the esophagus, as well as a bite of the esophagus itself. When taking the esophageal bite, it is important to avoid the anterior vagus nerve. Anchoring the wrap to the esophagus helps prevent slippage of the wrap, which is an important cause for failure of the operation.
- The fundoplication sutures are placed 1 cm apart, with the superior suture seated 2 cm above the GE junction and the inferior suture placed at the GE junction. The final wrap, then, is 2 cm in length (Figure 4-8).

Step 4. Postoperative Care

Inpatient Management

- The Foley catheter is removed at the end of the procedure.
- Patients are started on an aggressive antiemetic regimen in order to avoid retching, which can disrupt the crural repair and fundoplication.
- A liquid diet is started the night of the operation. The patient is advanced to a mechanical soft diet on the first postoperative day and discharged once he or she can tolerate the diet.

Postdischarge Management

- Patients remain on a soft diet for 3 to 4 weeks and then advance to a regular diet as tolerated.
- For the first 4 to 6 weeks after surgery, patients are counseled to avoid raw vegetables, tough meats, breads, and cakes.
- Patients who develop bloating should be counseled to eat smaller meals more frequently.
- For patients with dysphagia that fails to resolve by 6 to 8 weeks after surgery, endoscopic dilation should be considered.

Fundoplication

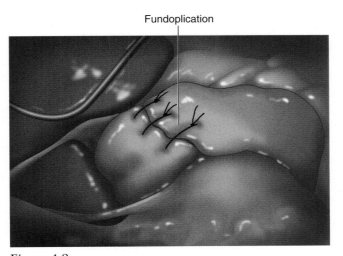

Figure 4-8

Step 5. Pearls and Pitfalls

- The key to success in antireflux surgery is patient selection. Operative candidates should have symptoms clearly attributable to reflux, as well as objective evidence of GERD.
- Upper endoscopy and esophageal manometry are essential studies prior to any antireflux operation, whereas 24-hour esophageal pH studies may be performed selectively.
- Full mobilization of the fundus is an important step to reduce the incidence of postoperative dysphagia.
- Mediastinal dissection should continue until a minimum of 2.5 cm to 3 cm of distal esophagus has been reduced into the abdomen.
- The fundoplication should be 2 cm in length and performed over a 56 French to 60 French dilator.
- A replaced or accessory left hepatic artery is present in up to 12% of patients and can be injured during dissection of the gastrohepatic ligament.
- The anterior and posterior vagus nerves must be identified and preserved from injury throughout the dissection to avoid the risk of gastroparesis.
- Energy use near the esophagus, particularly during the mediastinal dissection, is a potential source of unrecognized esophageal injury and should be kept to a minimum.
- The proximal short gastric vessels tear easily and should not be put under tension during mobilization of the fundus.

Selected References

Campos GM, Peters JH, DeMeester TR, et al: Multivariate analysis of factors predicting outcome after laparoscopic Nissen fundoplication. *J Gastrointest Surg* 3(3):292-300, 1999.

Fein M, Ritter MP, DeMeester TR, et al: Role of the lower esophageal sphincter and hiatal hernia in the pathogenesis of gastroesophageal reflux disease. *J Gastrointest Surg* 3(4):405-10, 1999.

Hunter JG, Swanstrom L, Waring JP: Dysphagia after laparoscopic antireflux surgery. The impact of operative technique. *Ann Surg* 224(1):51-57, 1996.

Hunter JG, Trus TL, Branum GD, et al: A physiologic approach to laparoscopic fundoplication for gastroesophageal reflux disease. *Ann Surg* 223(6):673-85, 1996.

Jobe BA, Kahrilas PJ, Vernon AH, et al: Endoscopic appraisal of the gastroesophageal valve after antireflux surgery. *Am J Gastroenterol* 99(2):233-43, 2004.

Mittal RK, Balaban DH: The esophagogastric junction. *NEJM* 336(13):924-32, 1997.

PARAESOPHAGEAL HERNIA

Ashley Haralson Vernon and Heidi L. Elliott

Step 1. Clinical Anatomy

- The main topic of this chapter is the operative management of paraesophageal hernias, which can also be referred to as giant hiatal hernias. These are usually managed by a surgeon and often require operative repair.
- Paraesophageal hernias (PEHs) are characterized by the migration of the gastroesophageal junction and the upper stomach into the mediastinum.
- There is typically a large anterior hernia sac that is composed of the attenuated phrenoesophageal ligament and two smaller posterior sacs. The sac is bordered by the mediastinal pleura, pericardium, and the aorta.
- The configuration of the stomach within the sac of a PEH may also be described in terms of its rotation, if present, in the organoaxial or mesioaxial position.

Step 2. Preoperative Considerations

- Patients often experience symptoms of heartburn and regurgitation because of the intrathoracic location of the gastroesophageal (GE) junction.
- Other frequently present symptoms include dysphagia, chest pain, and respiratory compromise, which are due to the mechanical effects of the herniated stomach in the mediastinum.
- The lining of the herniated stomach can develop deep ulcerations known as Cameron's ulcers, which may cause occult blood loss. Some patients may not have any gastrointestinal symptoms but suffer only from chronic anemia. It is not rare for the diagnosis of PEH to be made in the workup for iron deficiency anemia.
- Occasionally, one encounters a patient with a PEH who is truly asymptomatic. The classic teaching has been that these patients should undergo repair to avoid the chance of strangulation. Because of the rarity of this event, combined with the known risks associated with elective repair, most patients can be managed with watchful waiting.
- Most patients with PEH are intermittently symptomatic. These patients should undergo elective repair by a laparoscopic approach if there is no contraindication.
- In the rare event of strangulation of the herniated stomach, chest pain and foregut obstruction are the usual associated presenting signs. Treatment of this condition requires vigorous resuscitation and urgent laparotomy. Partial gastrectomy and reconstruction may be necessary.

Patient Preparation

- Patients with PEH need a broader preoperative evaluation than patients with GERD alone because they tend to be older and have more frequent cardiopulmonary conditions.
- In patients with significant preoperative nutritional deficiency or comorbidities that make operative repair too risky, endoscopic management may be best. One or sometimes two percutaneous gastrostomy tubes may provide gastric fixation and can also aid with postoperative nutrition.

Objective Testing

- A *barium swallow* can be used to assist in determining anatomy and operative planning.
- *Upper endoscopy* helps to identify mucosal erosions as a source of gastrointestinal bleeding and can rule out Barrett's esophagus and malignancy. This test should be attempted knowing that sometimes it is technically impossible to obtain.
- *Esophageal motility study* and *24-hour pH studies* are difficult to perform because they require intraesophageal positioning of the catheter or probe. Fortunately, the incidence of motility disorders is rare in this population, and there is no need to prove esophageal acid exposure before operating on the patient.
- *Pulmonary function tests* should be performed in patients with a history of shortness of breath or impaired exercise tolerance. Significant improvement in restrictive lung disease can be expected after surgery.

Equipment and Instrumentation

◆ The procedure is performed through five ports: three 5-mm ports and two 10-mm ports. The left upper quadrant 10-mm port can be upsized to accommodate a roticulating endo-scopic stapler if an esophageal lengthening procedure is to be performed.
◆ A 30-degree 10-mm laparoscope is used.
◆ A ¼-inch 4-cm long Penrose drain secured with a chromic Endoloop is useful for retracting the upper stomach.
◆ Advanced laparoscopic instruments are needed, including atraumatic bowel graspers such as Hunter graspers (Jarit), laparoscopic Metzenbaum scissors, and needle drivers.
◆ The hook electrocautery is fast and can be used for much of the dissection of the crura. The laparoscopic 5-mm curved harmonic scalpel (ultrasonic coagulator) is used for division of the short gastric vessels and mediastinal dissection.

Anesthesia

◆ Patients with severe carbon dioxide retention, noted during the preoperative workup, can be difficult to manage intraoperatively. The anesthesiologist can reduce CO_2 retention by increasing minute ventilation, and the surgeon can decrease the level of CO_2 absorption by decreasing the pneumoperitoneum. An alternative insufflating agent such as nitrous oxide can be used.
◆ Following induction of general anesthesia, an orogastric tube and Foley catheter are placed. If there is difficulty passing the orogastric tube, it should not be forced, but it should be attempted again after the contents of the sac have been reduced.

Room Setup and Patient Positioning

◆ The patient is placed supine on a split leg table with arms out and the legs abducted in a 45-degree angle at the hip. Footplates are used to prevent sliding when the patient is placed in reverse Trendelenburg position.
◆ The surgeon stands between the patient's legs to allow for the best access to the hiatus. The assistant stands on the patient's left side. Monitors are placed at the head of the table.

Step 3. Operative Steps

Access and Port Placement

- The abdomen is insufflated using a Veress needle at the umbilicus or in the left upper quadrant when a prior midline incision was made.
- The procedure is performed through five ports.
  - ▲ A 10-mm camera port is placed 15 cm below the xiphoid and just to the left of the midline to avoid the falciform ligament (Figure 5-1). This port needs to be high on the abdomen so that visualization into the mediastinum is possible if an extended mediastinal dissection is necessary (shortened esophagus).
  - ▲ The surgeon's right hand access is through a 10-mm port along the left costal margin, 12 cm from the xiphoid process.
  - ▲ A 5-mm port is placed in a right lateral position just off the costal margin for the liver retractor. Retraction of the left lobe of the liver to expose the hiatus can be achieved with a 5-mm "triangle" retractor, fixed to a flexible retractor arm "snake" mounted to the Book-walter post on the right side of the table. Alternatively, the Nathanson retractor can be placed through a 5-mm subxiphoid port and mounted from the left side.
  - ▲ The assistant uses a 5-mm port in the left flank, anterior axillary line, approximately 4 to 6 cm inferior to the surgeon's right-hand port.
  - ▲ The final port placed is a 5-mm port in the right upper abdomen for the surgeon's left hand access. It is placed just off the costal margin in the midclavicular line. This port needs to be as high as possible on the abdomen to reach up into the mediastinum. Its position is determined by the level of the liver.

Reduction of the Hernia

The hernia is reduced with the aid of gravity and gentle traction. The table is placed in steep reverse Trendelenburg, which does much of the work of retraction. The assistant retracts the herniated contents inferiorly, and the surgeon pulls the GE junction out of the mediastinum (Figure 5-2).

Different from a standard procedure fundoplication, the surgeon begins at the left crus of the diaphragm, not the right. The peritoneum overlying the abdominal side of the left crus is opened (Figure 5-3). The sac is then pulled inferiorly and medially out of the chest and away from the mediastinal pleura, which appears much whiter than the sac (Figure 5-4).

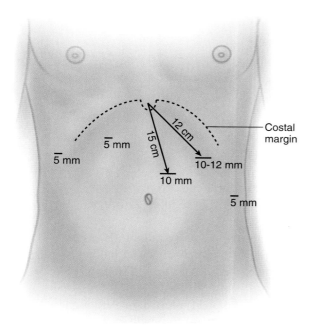

Figure 5-1

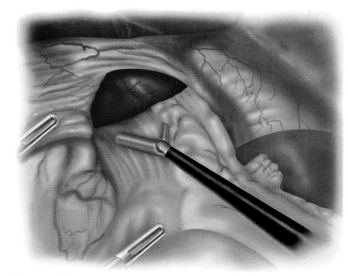

Figure 5-2

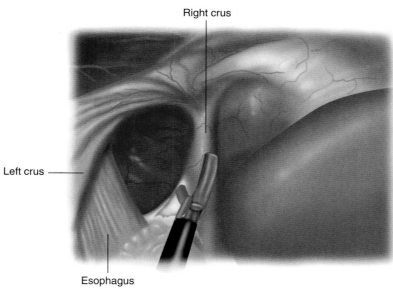

Figure 5-3

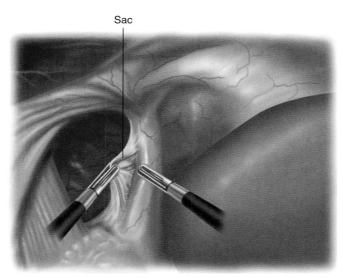

Figure 5-4

Excision of the Sac

- The dissection continues up and over the anterior aspect of the crural defect to expose the right crus (Figure 5-5). The assistant can hold the sac to prevent it from retracting into the chest.
- The sac will be attached to the mediastinum with filmy adhesions, which can be torn easily. If the tissue does not tear easily with two grasps, then you have probably encountered a blood vessel. The Harmonic scalpel should be used to provide hemostasis in addition to division (Figure 5-6).
- To remove the sac, it must be divided from the gastroesophageal fat pad (Figure 5-7). Although the inclination is to "clean off" the GE junction, it is, in fact, more prudent to divide the sac a fair distance away from the GE fat pad to avoid inadvertent injury to the anterior vagus. The anterior vagus can be displaced off of the esophagus because of the hernia.
- Mobilization of the fundus is necessary to facilitate the posterior dissection. The short gastric vessels (which are frequently quite long) are divided using the ultrasonic dissector. The surgeon retracts the stomach to the patient's right side, while the assistant retracts the short gastric vessels anteriorly and laterally. As you approach the top of the stomach where the vessels are shorter, the assistant can retract the posterior fundus ("behind" the short gastrics) to the patient's right side, which will tent the vessels and avoid thermal spread to the stomach wall.
- The posterior sac is then reduced and detached from the crura. It is not easily defined like the anterior sac. It is important that the posterior crura are cleared of attachments before suturing them closed.

Establishment of Adequate Intra-Abdominal Esophageal Length

- It is helpful to encircle the esophagus with a 4-cm long, ¼-inch wide Penrose drain secured with an Endoloop (Covidien, Mansfield, Massachusetts). The assistant retracts the esophagus to the patient's right, allowing visualization of the retroesophageal window, the left crus, and dissection can be continued if necessary. The posterior vagus is adjacent to the esophagus, wrapped within the Penrose drain.
- At least 2 cm of intra-abdominal esophagus below the level of the crura is necessary for completing the wrap. If there is inadequate length, an extensive mediastinal esophageal mobilization should be undertaken. This is usually all that is needed to obtain the needed length.

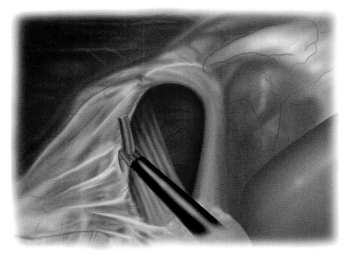

Figure 5-5

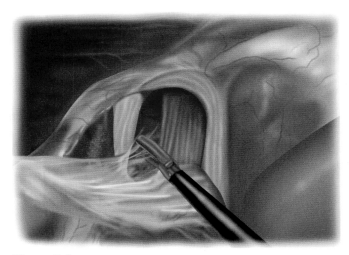

Figure 5-6

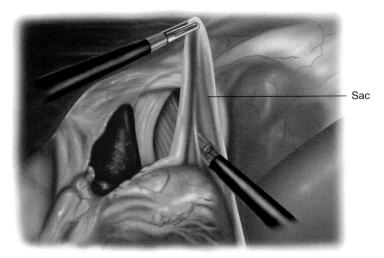

Sac

Figure 5-7

Closure of the Hiatal Defect

◆ The diaphragmatic defect is closed posteriorly with interrupted 0-silk, or 0-Ethibond (Ethicon, Somerville, New Jersey) suture, starting at the base of the crura. In large hernias, the crura often lack integrity and will need to be reinforced with pledgets.
◆ The pledgets should be sized so that they do not come in contact with the esophagus but lie exclusively on the crura (Figure 5-8).

Mesh Reinforcement

◆ Biologic mesh has been shown to reduce hernia recurrence when compared to primary repair. The mesh needs to be sutured to the diaphragm to prevent malpositioning.
◆ After the hiatus is closed posteriorly, a piece of mesh is fashioned in a U-shape and secured to the diaphragm using interrupted silk sutures. Placing spiral tacks in this area is discouraged, as there have been reports of penetration of the pericardium.

Fundoplication

◆ A fundoplication should be performed to both prevent postoperative reflux and provide further anchoring of the stomach and esophagus intra-abdominally.
◆ The fundus should be free to pass behind the esophagus without traction.
◆ A floppy 2-cm long 360-degree wrap is performed over a 56 to 60 Fr bougie. The fundoplication is secured using three 2-0 nonabsorbable sutures (silk or Ethibond). Each stitch should incorporate a full thickness of stomach and partial thickness of esophagus (Figure 5-9).
◆ The orogastric tube is then removed.

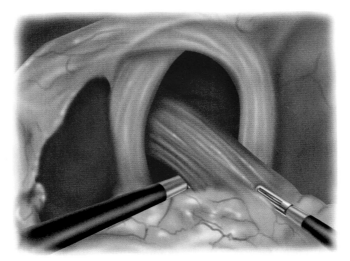

Figure 5-8

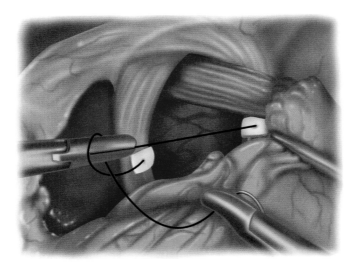

Figure 5-9

Collis Gastroplasty

In patients with shortened esophagus, a Collis gastroplasty should be performed.
- Extensive mediastinal mobilization at least 4 to 6 cm above the GE junction is carried out.
- The orogastric tube is replaced with a 48 Fr bougie, and a point 3 cm inferior to the angle of His, just lateral to the bougie, is marked with electrocautery.
- A roticulating 45-mm endoscopic stapler is introduced into the abdomen through the left subcostal port and fired transversely across the fundus until the marked point is reached.
- The stapler is then reloaded and fired parallel to the esophagus, abutting the bougie, so that a wedge of gastric fundus approximately 15 mL in volume is removed. This creates the neo-esophagus that is approximately 3 to 4 cm in length.
- After stapling is complete, the bougie is replaced with an orogastric tube, and 250 mL of methylene blue is used to fill the stomach and test the staple lines for leaks.

Gastropexy

- A gastropexy may help to prevent recurrent herniation of the stomach into the chest from constant positive intra-abdominal pressure or crural disruption.
- Two 0-Prolene sutures are placed in the midbody of the stomach in an area that will easily reach the anterior abdominal wall. Each tail is then brought out through the skin at two separate fascia puncture sites and secured.

Step 4. Postoperative Care

Inpatient Management

- Patients may begin liquids on the first postoperative day, or if extensive dissection was required, a contrast swallow study may be performed prior to starting a diet.
- Postoperative nausea is treated aggressively. For the first 24 hours postoperatively, patients are placed on around-the-clock antiemetic regimens.
- Patients are usually discharged on the second postoperative day on a full liquid diet.
- The diet is then advanced over the next few days to soft solid food. Patients remain on soft solids for 3 to 4 weeks.

Long-Term Management

- Patients are instructed to avoid breads, dry meats, and carbonated beverages.
- If the prescribed diet is followed, most patients will not complain of dysphagia. When symptoms are present with liquids or if solids are not tolerated after 3 to 4 weeks, then an upper gastrointestinal contrast study can be helpful. Ultimately, endoscopic dilation may be needed.
- Over the long term, many patients after surgery will have abnormalities found on upper gastrointestinal contrast studies; however, most of these patients are asymptomatic or minimally symptomatic.

Step 5. Pearls and Pitfalls

- An antireflux procedure should be performed on patients undergoing PEH repair because the majority of them will have abnormal 24-hr pH studies postoperatively without it.
- During the reduction of the hernia sac, constant attention to the location and preservation of the vagus nerves, esophagus, and aorta should be maintained. The vagus nerves should be identified and preserved to avoid postoperative gastroparesis.
- Complete sac mobilization and resection should be achieved.
- The most challenging aspect of a laparoscopic PEH repair is dissection of the inferior left crus. The key to achieving this is adequate esophageal mobilization and division of the short gastric vessels.
- Most cases of shortened esophagus are corrected with extensive mediastinal mobilization. This may eliminate the need for an esophageal lengthening procedure.
- If the mediastinal pleura is entered, laparoscopic dissection should continue unless the patient's condition deteriorates. Repair of the pleura can potentially create a dangerous flap that may lead to a tension pneumothorax.
- The use of prosthetic mesh at the hiatus introduces a potentially catastrophic outcome for patients: erosion into the esophagus. Biologic materials offer a safer and equally effective alternative for bolstering the crural repair.

Selected References

Low DE, Simchuk EJ: Effect of paraesophageal hernia repair on pulmonary function. *Ann Surg* 74:333-337, 2002.
Oelschlager BK, Pellegrini CA, Hunter J, et al: Biologic prosthesis reduces recurrence after lap paraesophageal hernia repair: a multi-center prospective randomized trial. *Ann Surg* 244(4):481-90, 2006.
Ponsky J, Rosen M, Fanning A, et al: Anterior gastropexy may reduce the recurrence rate after laparoscopic paraesophageal hernia repair. *Surg Endosc* 17(7):1036-41, 2003.
Stylopoulos N, Gazelle GS, Rattner DW: Paraesophageal hernias: operation or observation? *Ann Surg* 236(4):492-501, 2002.
Swanstrom LL, Marcus DR, Galloway GQ: Laparoscopic Collis gastroplasty is the treatment of choice for the shortened esophagus. *Am J Surg* 171(5):477-81, 1996.
Tsereteli Z, Terry ML, et al: Prospective randomized clinical trial comparing nitrous oxide and carbon dioxide pneumoperitoneum for laparoscopic surgery. *J Am Coll Surg* 195(2):173-9, 2002.

CHAPTER 6

GASTRIC WEDGE RESECTION

Chandrajit P. Raut

Step 1. Clinical Anatomy

- Gastric wedge resections may be performed for gastric tumors such as early gastric adenocarcinoma (lesions <25 mm in size), gastrointestinal stromal tumors, or other gastric tumors.
- Wedge resections to establish a diagnosis may be indicated if other less invasive diagnostic modalities have been unsuccessful.
- Wedge resections may also be performed for palliation of symptoms such as tumor hemorrhage for otherwise advanced, unresectable gastric neoplasms (for instance, in patients with distant metastatic disease).
- Tumors located at the GE junction or along the pyloric channel may not be appropriate for wedge resection because of the risk of luminal narrowing and may be more appropriately treated with conventional open or laparoscopic anatomic resections.
- Tumors along the lesser curvature may involve one or both vagus nerves. If both nerves are divided as part of the resection to achieve oncologically appropriate margins, pyloro-myotomy or pyloroplasty may be required.

Step 2. Preoperative Considerations

- The indications and contraindications for laparoscopic gastric wedge resections are similar to those for any open gastric resection.
- Patients who have had significant upper abdominal surgery with resulting dense adhesions may not be candidates for a laparoscopic approach, although a diagnostic laparoscopy may be performed at the beginning of the procedure to determine the feasibility of such an approach.

Patient Preparation

- Gastric tumors appropriate for wedge resection are generally identified either endoscopically or radiographically during workup of nonspecific upper abdominal symptoms, gastro-esophageal reflux, obstruction/early satiety, pain, or gastrointestinal hemorrhage.
- On upper endoscopy, tumors generally amenable to a laparoscopic wedge resection are submucosal lesions with an intact mucosal layer. Those that appear mucosal-based or ulcerated may not be appropriate for a wedge resection based on histologic diagnosis, and the planned approach should be reevaluated.
- On radiographic imaging, such as computed tomography (CT), tumors may appear as well-encapsulated or infiltrative lesions within the gastric wall or as exophytic lesions protruding intra- or extraluminally (Figure 6-1). Presence of extensive lymphadenopathy may suggest either lymphoma or gastric adenocarcinoma, necessitating a change in treatment.
- Additional imaging and laboratory studies for cancer staging may be ordered based on confirmed or suspected diagnosis.
- Endoscopic or image-guided fine-needle aspiration or core needle biopsy is indicated if the differential diagnosis would significantly change management. For instance, lymphoma would be treated with nonoperative, medical management, whereas gastric adenocarcinoma would require a more extensive gastric resection plus lymphadenectomy. Although resection for a gastric adenocarcinoma may also be performed laparoscopically, the resection involves removing more gastric tissue, and the procedure should be planned appropriately preoperatively.
- Some surgeons tattoo the lesion preoperatively, to assist in localization.

Equipment and Instrumentation

- Standard laparoscopic instruments may be used for gastric wedge resections:
  - ▲ 5-mm and 10-mm 30-degree video laparoscopes
  - ▲ Liver retractor
  - ▲ Harmonic scalpel (Ethicon, Somerville, New Jersey) or LigaSure (ValleyLab) for omental dissection, division of short gastric vessels, and adhesiolysis
  - ▲ Laparoscopic stapler
  - ▲ Specimen bag
  - ▲ Split leg table
- Intraoperative esophagogastroduodenoscopy may be helpful to localize the lesion, particularly for submucosal lesions, which may not be readily visible laparoscopically.

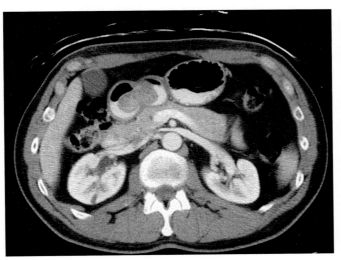

Figure 6-1

Anesthesia

- Procedures are performed under general anesthesia with muscle relaxant.
- Epidural anesthesia is not usually required.
- Topical anesthetic agents, such as 0.25% bupivacaine hydrochloride, may be infiltrated at each trocar site.
- At induction, intravenous antibiotics (generally a cephalosporin) are administered.
- A nasogastric tube and urinary catheter are inserted.

Room Setup and Patient Positioning

- A split-leg table may be helpful, allowing the primary surgeon to stand between the legs. The first assistant surgeon may stand on one side of the patient; a second assistant may stand on the opposite side. The scrub nurse/technician may stand opposite the first assistant or adjacent to either leg (Figure 6-2).
- Arms may be tucked or extended on arm boards at the discretion of the surgeon.
- If a single video monitor mounted from the ceiling is used, it may be positioned at the head of the table directly over the patient's head, allowing the surgeon standing between the legs to look directly ahead. If multiple monitors are used, either ceiling mounted or cart based, they may be placed on either side of the patient above the armboards.
- An endoscopy cart may be placed near the head of the operating table.

Step 3. Operative Steps

Access and Port Placement

- Pneumoperitoneum may be established using an open technique (at the site where the specimen will be extracted) or by insufflation via a Veress needle in the left upper quadrant at the discretion of the surgeon.
- Once pneumoperitoneum is established, four or five trocars may be placed in the upper abdomen.
- A 12-mm trocar placed supraumbilically midline or just left of midline will accommodate the stapler and specimen bag during the procedure.
- A port accommodating the liver retractor may be placed in the right upper quadrant, approximately 45 degrees off of midline and 12 cm to 15 cm from the xiphoid process. For lesions along the greater curvature of the midbody of the stomach well to the left of the lateral edge of the liver, or for instances where the left lateral segment of the liver is small, a liver retractor may not be necessary.
- Additional two or three 5-mm ports may be placed in the right and left upper quadrants for the dissecting and grasping instruments. These port sites may be upsized to 10 mm or 12 mm as needed to assist with placement of stapler or specimen bag, depending on the specific location of the tumor on the stomach (Figure 6-2).

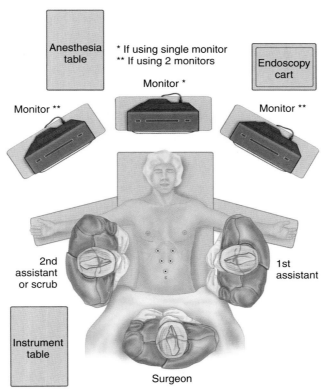

Figure 6-2

Mobilization

- The operating room table is repositioned in steep reverse Trendelenburg, allowing omentum and bowel to fall into the lower quadrants and out of the operative field.
- The abdomen is surveyed with the laparoscope in the supraumbilical port to identify the primary tumor site, evaluate for evidence of metastatic spread, and select the appropriate sites for the additional ports.
- Dissection of the greater and lesser curvatures of the stomach is performed selectively depending on the location of the tumor. The surgeon should avoid directly grasping or manipulating the tumor.
- For lesions close to the greater curvature, the omentum is carefully dissected away (the omentum does not necessarily have to be resected with the specimen for nonadenocarcinoma neoplasms). The greater curvature is grasped with a smooth grasper or Babcock clamp and retracted anteriorly (Figure 6-3). Counter traction may be placed directly on the omentum or on the transverse colon. The omentum is dissected off of the stomach using electrocautery, Harmonic scalpel, LigaSure, laparoscopic coagulating shears, or another dissecting instrument. Large branches of the gastroepiploic and short gastric vessels may be secured with clips. The spleen and splenic vessels are preserved.
- For lesions close to the lesser curvature, the gastrohepatic ligament is similarly divided. Branches of the right and left gastric vessels are divided between clips. The vagus nerves are preserved unless directly involved with the tumor.
- Adhesions in the lesser sac are carefully lysed.
- To avoid direct manipulation of the tumor, traction sutures may be placed proximal and distal (or anterior and posterior) to the tumor (Figure 6-4). These sutures may then be grasped for further manipulation rather than grasping the stomach itself.

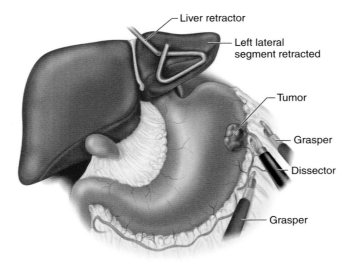

Liver retractor

Left lateral
segment retracted

Tumor

Grasper

Dissector

Grasper

Figure 6-3

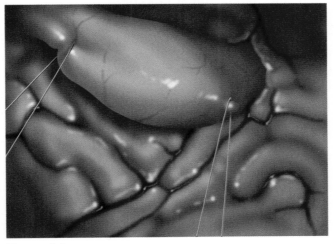

Figure 6-4

Division of Stomach

- Once the tumor has been sufficiently mobilized, an angulated stapler may be applied. One or more of the 5-mm ports may be upsized to a 12-mm port to accommodate the stapler as needed (Figure 6-5). The stapler should be applied such that the tumor plus a segment of normal surrounding stomach are removed as a wedge. This commonly requires sequential firings of the stapler.
- It is critical that a rim of normal stomach, measuring at least 1 cm, around the tumor is removed along with the tumor itself. If there is any concern about the margins of the tumor, an esophagogastroduodenoscopy should be performed to help identify the tumor edges, thereby preventing transection of the tumor. Gastric adenocarcinomas require a wider margin of resection, and thus the wedge resection described in this chapter is not appropriate for this latter diagnosis.
- The nasogastric tube should be withdrawn into the esophagus to eliminate the risk of it getting caught in the stapler.

Removal of Specimen and Completion of Procedure

- The gastric specimen, once freed, should be placed into a specimen bag.
- The gastric staple line should be inspected to rule out bleeding or leakage. Pinpoint sites of bleeding may be carefully cauterized or oversewn. If there is any concern of leakage, an esophagogastroduodenoscopy may be performed after filling the abdomen with saline (and taking the bed out of Trendelenburg position). Insufflation during endoscopy will test the integrity of the staple line. Bubbles from the staple line indicate a leak. The site must be repaired or oversewn. If necessary, the procedure may need to be converted to a laparotomy.
- The specimen may be extracted, which may require enlarging the port site. The specimen must be sent to pathology for immediate frozen section analysis to check the adequacy of the margins.
- The nasogastric tube should be repositioned in the stomach under visualization prior to removal of the ports.
- Larger fascial incisions should be reapproximated with sutures of the surgeon's choosing.
- Subcuticular dissolvable sutures may be used to close the skin incisions.

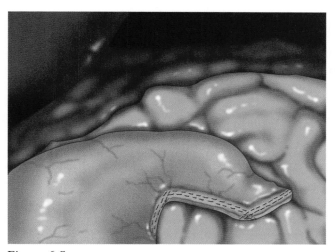

Figure 6-5

Step 4. Postoperative Care

- ◆ The nasogastric tube may be removed on postoperative day 1.
- ◆ Fluids may be started on postoperative day 2.
- ◆ Diet may be advanced at the discretion of the surgeon.

Step 5. Pearls and Pitfalls

- ◆ Oncologic principles must be maintained for gastric wedge resections performed for neoplasms. Margins of resection in the specimen must be evaluated by intraoperative frozen section analysis. The presence of tumor tissue at any margin of resection on frozen section analysis mandates reexcision at that time to achieve negative margins. The oncologic principles of tumor resection must not be compromised just to avoid a larger resection or conversion to a laparotomy.
- ◆ Some investigators have suggested that for patients undergoing partial gastric resections for tumors such as gastrointestinal stromal tumors, wedge gastrectomies may only be feasible for tumors localized to the fundus and greater curvature.
- ◆ Tumors in the antrum may require a laparoscopic distal gastrectomy, and those along the lesser curvature or near the gastroesophageal junction may require a laparoscopic transgastric resection. This is not consistently true. Ultimately, surgeons should determine which approach provides an adequate residual lumen and oncologically appropriate margin.

Selected References

Kitano S, Shiraishi N: Minimally invasive surgery for gastric tumors. *Surg Clin North Am* 85(1): 151-64, xi, 2005.
Ohgami M, Otani Y, Furukawa T, et al: Curative laparoscopic surgery for early gastric cancer: eight years experience. *Nihon Geka Gakkai Zasshi* 101(8):539-45, 2000.
Otani Y, Ohgami M, Igarashi N, et al: Laparoscopic wedge resection of gastric submucosal tumors. *Surg Laparosc Endosc Percutan Tech* 10(1):19-23, 2000.
Privette A, McCahill L, Borrazzo E, et al: Laparoscopic approaches to resection of suspected gastric gastrointestinal stromal tumors based on tumor location. *Surg Endosc* 22(2):487-494, 2008.

PEPTIC ULCER SURGERY

Gregory J. Mancini and Matthew L. Mancini

Step 1. Surgical Anatomy

- A dissection of the esophagus at the hiatus will expose the anterior and posterior vagal trunks.
- The anterior vagus is intimately related to the anterior esophagus as it traverses from left to right. Circumferential dissection of the vagal trunk will permit placement of surgical clips as well as interval truncal resection for pathologic confirmation.
- The posterior vagal trunk has a more variable association to the esophagus but is most often found along the right esophagus between the 7 and 9 o'clock position.
- When performing an antrectomy, the gastroduodenal artery should be ligated to ensure proper mobilization of the first and second portion of the duodenum.
- The chronic regional inflammation may hinder dissection of the pylorus from the head of the pancreas.
- Inadequate mobilization could impair stapling distal to the pylorus and leave retained antrum at the staple line. Retained antrum may lead to recurrent ulcer disease and surgical failure. A full Kocher maneuver is rarely necessary to achieve adequate duodenal mobilization.

Step 2. Preoperative Considerations

Patient Preparation

- The advent of proton pump inhibitors (PPIs) has greatly diminished the frequency and volume of peptic ulcer surgery for the practicing general surgeon. Conversely, because of the use and availability of PPIs, only the most severe cases of ulcer disease present for surgical evaluation. A cautious and thorough preoperative workup is paramount.

- Patient selection may be the most difficult preoperative activity for the physician. PPI medication noncompliance, chronic NSAID use, smoking, and alcohol use are the most common patient factors that aggravate the disease process. Likewise, these patient factors predict poorer clinical outcomes from surgical intervention. All patients should be counseled appropriately.
- The ubiquity of proton pump inhibitors (PPIs) has greatly impacted the frequency and volume of peptic ulcer surgery. Additionally, advancements in therapeutic endoscopic techniques, such as pneumatic balloon dilatation, have reduced the need for the classically described antiulcer surgical procedures. Though the frequency of antiulcer operations has dropped, the severity of ulcer disease that prevails often yields the need for surgical evaluation.
- The most common indication for vagotomy and pyloroplasty is gastric outlet obstruction caused by chronic and recurring pyloric channel ulcer disease. Most patients will have had one or multiple therapeutic endoscopic procedures, such as pneumatic balloon dilatation. Reviewing the endoscopic procedure history and photographic documentation will enhance not only correct patient selection but also correct procedural selection.
- The most common indication for vagotomy and antrectomy is a chronic nonhealing peptic ulcer. In addition to removing any concerning gastric pathology, antrectomy will also improve acid suppression. Depending on the indication, the antrectomy may improve acid suppression and/or remove concerning gastric pathology. Prior to surgical evaluation, patients may have had months of multidrug antiulcer therapy, repeated H. pylori eradication regimens, and numerous ulcer biopsies to rule out occult malignancy. Reviewing the endoscopic procedure history, biopsy pathology results, and procedural photographic documentation will enhance both patient selection and correct procedural selection.

Anesthesia

- General endotracheal intubation is recommended for this procedure. The anesthesiologist may insert an orogastric tube to decompress the stomach after induction. Your anesthesia team may prefer a rapid sequence protocol because of the aspiration risk associated with retained gastric contents. Alternatively, if endoscopy is planned as an adjunct to the laparoscopic procedure, therapeutic endoscopic suction and decompression after intubation would be advantageous.

Room Setup and Patient Positioning

- Patients are positioned in supine position with arms out and secured on arm boards. A footboard is secured at the end of the bed to maintain proper patient safety when placed in the reverse Trendelenburg position.

Step 3. Operative Steps

Truncal Vagotomy with Pyloroplasty

Access and Port Placement

- Combining the truncal vagotomy with pyloroplasty makes port site placement different from most other foregut operations. The inferior and right lateral location of the pylorus requires moving the camera and surgeon's working ports to a more inferior position on the abdomen.
- The location for optimal triangulation of the pylorus can be achieved by placing the three trocars in line at the level of the umbilicus. A fourth trocar can be placed in the left subcostal location for an assistant's instrument. A liver retractor, such as a Nathanson retractor, can be placed though a subxyphoid access site.

Truncal Vagotomy

- The truncal vagotomy can be performed early in the operation, and often as the first step. Begin by opening the pars flaccida of the gastrohepatic ligament to facilitate identification of the right crus. Division of the phrenoesophageal ligament anterior to the esophagus will permit entry into the mediastinum. A limited dissection of the esophagus at the hiatus will expose the anterior and posterior vagal trunks.
- Circumferential dissection of the vagal trunks will permit placement of proximal and distal surgical clips as well as interval truncal resection for pathologic confirmation.
- Anterior vagotomy (Figure 7-1).
- Posterior vagotomy (Figure 7-2).

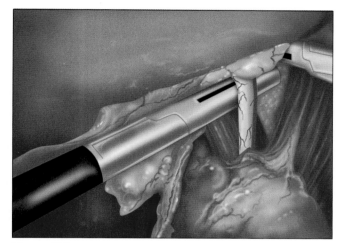

Figure 7-1

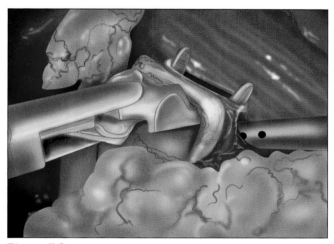

Figure 7-2

Pyloroplasty

- When addressing the pyloroplasty, expect adhesions to the omentum and gallbladder overlying the duodenum resulting from the chronic inflammatory process.
- Placement of a superior and inferior traction suture facilitates optimal exposure and control of the tissue. A generous transverse incision should be extending 2 to 3 cm on both sides of the pylorus. The fibrotic and often circumferential nature of this lesion makes the closure difficult. Extending the incision onto soft, pliable tissue of both the antrum and duodenum makes the laparoscopic closure easier. A 4- to 6-cm pyloroplasty should be performed. The longer pyloroplasty will create a larger cross-sectional area that will reduce the risk of postoperative stenosis (Figure 7-3a).
- It is important to open the ulcer channel between the antral and duodenal sides of the pylorus. This channel can be short or long, but it is typically very sclerotic and narrow. Endoscopic placement of a transpyloric feeding tube or guidewire greatly facilitates guidance of the enterotomy across the pyloric channel (Figure 7-3b).
- Laparoscopic vertical closure of the pyloroplasty is accomplished by a running single full-thickness closure, a Heineke-Mikulicz pyloroplasty. To ensure closure of the incision's corners, begin separate sutures at the superior and inferior corners, meeting in the center (Figure 7-3c).
- Once the pyloroplasty is closed, endoscopic visualization confirms both the patency of the lumen and air tightness of the sutured repair.

Closing

- The fascia of 10-mm port sites are closed per physician routine. Skin site closure is completed using 5-0 absorbable suture in subcuticular fashion.

Laparoscopic Truncal Vagotomy with Antrectomy with Billroth II Anastomosis

Access and Port Placement

- Trocar positioning for this operation is similar to most foregut operations. A camera port placed 15 cm below the xyphoid process will optimize the view of stomach, the ligament of Treitz, and the esophageal hiatus. Two ports are inserted for the surgeon on the right side of the upper abdomen. A left subcostal trocar will allow an assistant to provide proper retraction. A liver retractor, such as a Nathanson retractor, can be placed though a subxyphoid access site.

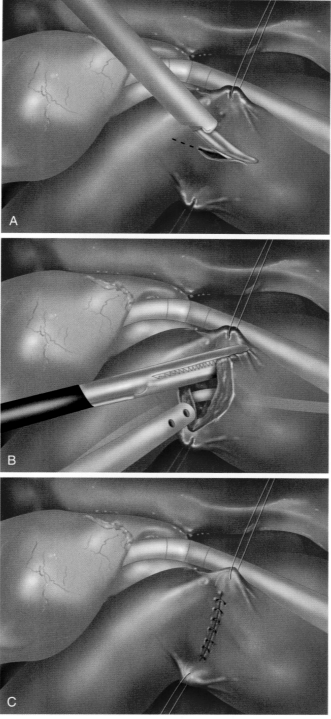

Figure 7-3

See the preceding information for details of truncal vagotomy.

Antrectomy

- Proceeding to the antrectomy, the lesser sac is entered along the greater curvature of the stomach. The dissection is carried toward the pylorus and behind the stomach to its lesser curve (Figure 7-4).
- The gastroduodenal artery will be ligated to ensure adequate duodenal mobilization.
- Next, the dissection is started along the stomach's lesser curvature and the superior margin of the duodenum's second portion.
- A full Kocher maneuver is rarely necessary to achieve adequate duodenal mobilization, although mobilization of the first and second portion of the duodenum is important. The chronic regional inflammation may hinder dissection of the pylorus from the head of the pancreas. Inadequate mobilization could impair proper stapling distal to the pylorus and thereby create a problem of retained antrum. Retained antrum may lead to recurrent ulcer disease and surgical failure.
- Once mobile, the duodenum is divided using a linear laparoscopic stapling device (Figure 7-5).
- A linear transection line across the stomach is chosen to ensure removal of the antrum. Once the antrectomy is complete, the specimen is set aside for removal at the end of the procedure.

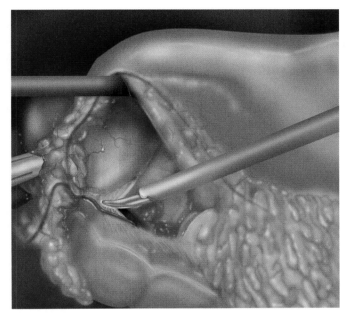

Figure 7-4

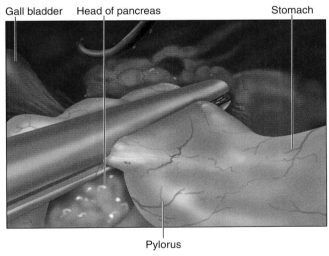

Figure 7-5

Billroth II Anastomosis

- The gastrojejunal anastomosis begins by identifying the proximal jejunum. The ligament of Treitz is identified by elevating the greater omentum and transverse colon. Next, a window is made through the transverse mesocolon just above the ligament of Treitz (Figure 7-6).
- The proximal jejunum is placed through the mesocolon window and pulled through into the lesser sac. This creates a retrocolic orientation of the gastrojejunostomy.
- Next, a side-to-side, functional end-to-side gastrojejunostomy is created using a laparoscopic linear stapling device (Figure 7-7).
- The common enterotomy created with this technique is closed laparoscopically with a running single-layer sutured closure.
- Creation of the gastrojejunostomy can be performed in either a retrocolic or antecolic fashion. The benefit to the retrocolic position is the ability to bring the jejunum directly from the fixed position at the ligament of Treitz to the gastric staple line. This creates the shortest afferent limb, minimizing the risk of afferent limb syndrome postoperatively.

Closing

- The fascia of 10-millimeter port sites are closed per physician routine. Skin site closure is completed using 5-0 absorbable suture in subcuticular fashion.

Step 4. Postoperative Care

- The patient is kept NPO (nil per os) until a Gastrografin upper gastrointestinal swallow study is complete. This study documents patency of the intestinal lumen and competency of closure.
- A strict postoperative diet, beginning with clear liquids and advancing to a solid diet over a 6-week period, may allow for proper intestinal healing and mitigate patient dietary intolerances.
- Reinforcement of the importance of good patient lifestyle choices, mainly smoking cessation, NSAID cessation alcohol abstinence, and PPI medication compliance, will enhance patient outcomes.

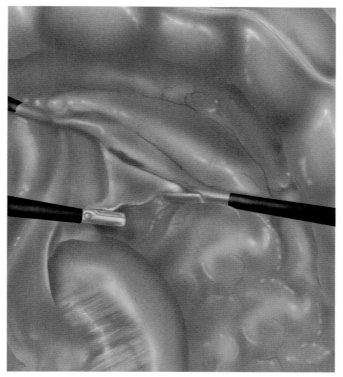

Figure 7-6

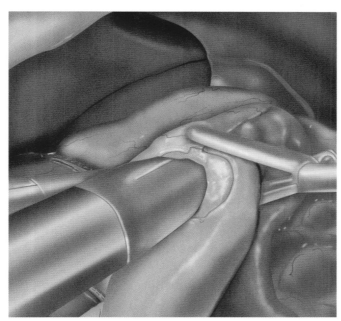

Figure 7-7

Step 5. Pearls and Pitfalls

- Patient selection and preoperative preparation stresses the positive impact that healthy lifestyle choices will improve long-term outcomes. The procedure emphasizes the importance of smoking cessation, alcohol abstinence, and that PPI medication compliance is paramount.
- The value of intraoperative endoscopy cannot be over emphasized.
  - ▲ At the beginning of the case, decompressing the stomach will limit the aspiration risk at the time of extubation.
  - ▲ Endoscopic placement of a feeding tube or guidewire across the stenotic pyloric channel will assist properly traversing the lesion and avoid back wall injury to the duodenum that could fistulize or leak.
  - ▲ Additionally, passage of an adult endoscope (1.5 cm in diameter) across the closure site validates the patency of the lumen.

Acute Peptic Ulcer Perforation

Step 1. Surgical Anatomy

- In emergency surgery such as perforated peptic ulcer disease, the difficulty identifying the pertinent anatomy depends greatly on the duration and severity of the perforation.
- The majority of perforations presenting emergently will occur on the anterior stomach and duodenum. Entering the lesser sac along the greater curve will facilitate posterior wall inspection.

Step 2. Preoperative Considerations

- Despite the widespread use of prescription PPIs and over-the-counter H2 blocker medications, peptic ulcer disease remains one of the most common causes of acute intestinal perforation requiring emergent surgical treatment. Smoking, alcohol use, and medication non-compliance are common patient factors contributing to disease prevalence. Additionally, the rise in chronic use of over-the-counter non-steroidal anti-inflammatory drugs (NSAIDs) has, in particular, elevated the risk of ulcer perforation.
- The traditional treatment has been and remains: preoperative volume resuscitation of the patient, surgical treatment including washout and source control, and diligent postoperative care. Over the last two decades the primary method of source control has been omental patching of the perforated ulcer (Graham patch). Additionally, ulcer resection may be used for gastric ulcers on mobile portions of the stomach.
- The use of laparoscopic techniques in cases of acute intestinal perforation is an emerging area for application. Though several cases series in the 1990s proved the safety and efficacy of minimally invasive techniques, in 2008 less than 5% of all cases of perforated peptic ulcers were treated laparoscopically.

Anesthesia

- Positioning
- See the earlier discussion

Step 3. Operative Steps

Access and Port Placement

- Trocar positioning for this operation is similar to laparoscopic pyloroplasty procedure. A camera port placed 15 cm below the xyphoid process will optimize the view of the entire abdomen. The location for optimal triangulation of the pylorus can be achieved by placing the three trocars in line at the level of the umbilicus.
- A fourth trocar can be placed in the left subcostal location for an assistant's instrument. A liver retractor, such as a Nathanson retractor, can be placed though a subxyphoid access site.
- Once laparoscopic access has been achieved, a careful inspection of the abdomen is performed, making special note of loculated fluid collections that will require thorough irrigation.

- Next, localization of the perforation site is carried out. Anterior perforations of the stomach and duodenum are most common, but locating the perforation may be or prove difficult. Intra-operative endoscopy can facilitate the search. If not directly visualized endoscopically, the insufflation of air to distend the stomach will force air through the perforation creating a bubbling effect seen laparoscopically.
- Once located, a thorough irrigation and inspection is done to fully evaluate the location, size, and depth of the ulcer.
- In the case of an ulcer occurring on the body of the stomach, laparoscopic ulcer resection can be considered. This should be a full-thickness gastric wall resection and can be potentially done as a stapled resection. Placement of stay sutures along the ulcer edge can assist in ensuring proper laparoscopic stapler positioning (Figure 7-8).
- For ulcers on the lesser curve of the stomach or pylorus, resection is unlikely. A Graham patch procedure can be performed laparoscopically. A pedicle of omentum is needed for the laparoscopic Graham patch. Dividing the omentum vertically up to the transverse colon creates a long free pedicle of omentum that can reach without tension.
- Next, 3 to 5 sutures are placed taking seromuscular bites on both sides of the ulcer. The omental pedicle is placed over the ulcer and on top of the sutures. Sequential tying of the interrupted sutures is completed securing the Graham patch (Figure 7-8).
- An air leak test can be performed by endoscopically insufflating the stomach while irrigating the repair.
- Gastric ulcers should either be biopsied to rule out malignancy, or resected if located on a mobile portion of the stomach. The laparoscopic Graham patch may be completed after biopsy or resection similar to the manner described above.
- After source control is complete, thorough washout of the abdomen and pelvis should be done. By repositioning the bed from right to left and from head up to head down, copious irrigation can be accomplished, thereby removing contamination.

Closing

- The fascia of 10 mm trocar sites are closed per physician routine. Skin site closure is completed using 5-0 absorbable suture in subcuticular fashion.

Step 4. Postoperative Care

- Postoperative treatment for Helicobacter pylori and PPI therapy is recommended, even if pathology or serology is negative.

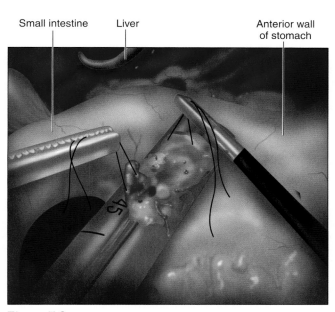

Figure 7-8

Step 5. Pearls and Pitfalls

- The primary failure rate of the Graham patch procedure has been reported to be between 5% and 25%. This has not changed with laparoscopic techniques. An omental pedicle flap secured under tension may be one reason for Graham patch leakage. Dividing the greater omentum vertical up to the transverse colon will yield a pedicle that will reach without tension and preserve omental pedicle perfusion.
- A second potential factor for patch failure may be related to suture fixation techniques of the pedicle. Common leakage points are at the superior or inferior margins of the ulcer-patch repair. Placing fixation sutures above and below the ulcer margins will reduce the chance of leakage from the apical margins of the Graham patch repair.
- Management of 3 to 5 intracorporeal sutures at one time can be cumbersome. Using two different suture materials or colors, for instance 2-0 silk and 2-0 Vicryl, may make intracorporeal knot-tying and omental pedicle fixation less frustrating.

Selected References

Arora G, Singh G, Triadafilopoulos G: Proton pump inhibitors for gastroduodenal damage related to nonsteroidal anti-inflammatory drugs or aspirin: twelve important questions for clinical practice. *Clin Gastroenterol Hepatol* 7(7):725-35, 2009.

Bertleff MJ, Halm JA, Bemelman WA, et al: Randomized clinical trial of laparoscopic versus open repair of the perforated peptic ulcer: the LAMA Trial. *World J of Surg* 33(7):1368-73, 2009.

Fromm D, Resitarits D, Kozol R: An analysis of when patients eat after gastrojejunostomy. *Ann Surg* 207(1):14-20,1988.

Gutiérrez de la Peña C, Márquez R, Fakih F, et al: Simple closure or vagotomy and pyloroplasty for the treatment of a perforated duodenal ulcer: comparison of results. *Dig Surg* 17(3):225-28, 2000.

Gibson JB, Behrman SW, Fabian TC, Britt LG: Gastric outlet obstruction resulting from peptic ulcer disease requiring surgical intervention is infrequently associated with Helicobacter pylori infection. *J Am Coll Surg* 191(1):32-37, 2000.

Hermansson M, Ekedahl A, Ranstam J, Zilling T: Decreasing incidence of peptic ulcer complications after the introduction of the proton pump inhibitors, a study of the Swedish population from 1974-2002. *BMC Gastroenterol* (9):25, 2009.

Hobsley M, Tovey FI, Holton J: Precise role of H pylori in duodenal ulceration. *World J Gastroenterol* 12(40):6413-19, 2006.

Laws HL, McKernan JB: Endoscopic management of peptic ulcer disease. *Ann Surg* 217(5):548-55,1993.

Matsuda M, Nishiyama M, Hanai T, et al: Laparoscopic omental patch repair for perforated peptic ulcer. *Ann Surg* 221(3):236-40, 1995.

Mihmanli M, Isgor A, Kabukcuoglu F, et al: The effect of H. pylori in perforation of duodenal ulcer. *Hepatogastroenterology* 45(23): 1610-12, 1998.

Rivera RE, Eagon JC, Soper NJ, et al: Experience with laparoscopic gastric resection: results and outcomes for 37 cases. *Surg Endosc* 19(12):1622-26, 2005.

Sachdeva K, Zaren HA, Sigel B: A Surgical treatment of peptic ulcer disease. *Med Clin North Am* 75(4):999-1012, 1991.

Søreide, K, Sarr, MG, Søreide, JA: Pyloroplasty for benign gastric outlet obstruction: indications and techniques. *Scand J Surg* 95(1): 11-16, 2006.

Vonkeman HE, Klok RM, Postma MJ, et al: Direct medical costs of serious gastrointestinal ulcers among users of NSAIDs. *Drugs Aging* 24(8):681-90, 2007.

Woodward ER: The history of vagotomy. *Am J Surg* 153(1):9-17, 1987.

CHAPTER 8

CHOLECYSTECTOMY

Ashley H. Vernon

Step 1. Surgical Anatomy

- The triangle of Calot is the most important anatomic boundary that needs to be defined when performing cholecystectomy. It is formed by the boundaries of the cystic duct, common hepatic duct, and cystic artery.
- Roughly parallel to this triangle is the hepatocystic triangle in which the cystic artery boundary is replaced with the liver edge. The only structure that should be found within this triangle is the cystic artery.

Step 2. Preoperative Considerations

Patient Preparation

- Straightforward symptoms of biliary colic along with objective evidence of gallstones by any imaging modality (ultrasound most sensitive) constitute adequate information to recommend cholecystectomy.
- In the absence of stones or sludge, studies of biliary function may help to diagnose pathology and need for surgery.
- Asymptomatic patients with stones do not generally require surgery unless immunocompromised. Obviously, the risks and benefits need to be weighed for each patient in making a recommendation for surgery.
- In cases of acute cholecystitis, inflammation of the gallbladder and bile ducts makes both open and laparoscopic cholecystectomy more difficult. In early or mild cases, the procedure can usually be managed laparoscopically. However, in severe cases it is often best to manage conservatively with intravenous antibiotics and delay surgery until the inflammation has subsided. Occasionally, in very sick patients, a cholecystostomy tube for drainage is also needed.

Equipment and Instrumentation

- ◆ A 30-degree scope is helpful for providing additional views, especially of the hepatocystic triangle and surrounding structures. Frequently the common bile duct can be seen without any dissection using this type of endoscope.
- ◆ Standard laparoscopic equipment is used, including the following:
  - ▲ Locking grasper to secure the fundus of the gallbladder
  - ▲ Atraumatic bowel grasper to maneuver the gallbladder infundibulum
  - ▲ Hand-operated L hook (attached to Bovie pencil) to perform dissection of the hepato-cystic triangle
  - ▲ Maryland dissector or a laparoscopic peanut to isolate the cystic duct and artery
  - ▲ Scissors, either Metzenbaum or guillotine, to transect the duct after clipping
- ◆ A clip applier is necessary to control the cystic duct. If the cystic duct is too large for a clip, then a pretied loop can be used to occlude the cystic duct stump.
- ◆ A specimen retrieval bag is recommended to prevent spillage of bile and stones into the abdomen during extraction of the gallbladder from the abdomen.

Anesthesia

- Prophylaxis for DVT is important in all patients undergoing laparoscopic procedures. We use sequential compression devices and subcutaneous heparin is started before induction with anesthesia.
- An orogastric tube is placed to decompress the stomach and duodenum to facilitate exposure during the procedure.
- Patients are asked to void before being brought to the operating room for their comfort after surgery. A Foley catheter is not usually necessary because ports are not placed in the lower abdomen. If a longer procedure is anticipated, then a catheter is placed at the beginning of the procedure.

Room Setup and Patient Positioning

- The patient is placed in the supine position. The surgeon operates from patient's left side. The arms may remain out on armboards unless a cholangiogram is anticipated, in which case the right arm should be tucked to make room for the C-arm.
- Although not usually an issue with thin patients, footplates are used to secure the patient on the table and prevent sliding, as most of the procedure is performed with the patient in the reverse Trendelenburg position.
- The table is rolled toward the left so that the abdominal contents fall into the left lower quadrant by gravity. This position is also more comfortable because the patient is brought closer to the surgeon and the left-handed instrument can reach the working port more easily.

Step 3. Operative Steps

Access and Port Placement

- The abdomen is insufflated using a Veress needle at the umbilicus, and a 10-mm port is placed through a vertical incision through the umbilicus. This allows the largest incision to be "hidden" entirely, as the scar will be buried in the base of the umbilicus (Figure 8-1).
- A 5-mm port is placed in the right flank, near the costal margin and lateral, just anterior to the right colon, so that it does not interfere with the operating surgeon's left hand. This is at the anterior axillary line. Through this port, the locking grasper is placed for retraction of the gallbladder fundus up and over the liver edge. It remains relatively stationary throughout the procedure.
- The upper epigastric port is used for introduction of the clip applier and must be at least 10 mm in size. The surgeon may choose to orient this in line with a subcostal incision in the event of a conversion to an open procedure. The surgeon's left-hand instruments are placed through a 5-mm port in the patient's right upper abdomen. It is optimal if the camera and two operating ports form a diamond shape with the gallbladder at the top corner. The assistant will hold the camera and direct the retraction of the gallbladder fundus.
- The procedure is performed through four ports. To prevent port site hernias, try to use the smallest ports possible for the procedure. For most patients, opt to use two 10-mm ports—one for the 10-mm scope and the other for the 10-mm clip applier. By using a 5-mm scope and a 5-mm clip applier, the procedure can be accomplished using all small instruments, although one port, usually the umbilical port, will need to be enlarged to remove the gallbladder.

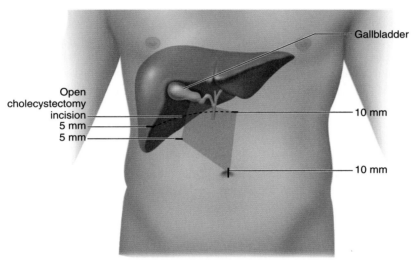

Gallbladder

Open
cholecystectomy
incision

5 mm

5 mm

10 mm

10 mm

Figure 8-1

Description of Procedure

- The operation begins by exposing the gallbladder infundibulum. The assistant gently retracts the fundus in a cephalad direction, bringing the entire length of the gallbladder into view. Often, adhesions to the upper part of the gallbladder prevent this maneuver and must be divided using the hook electrocautery or stripped away from the gallbladder bluntly.
- Once retraction is secured, the patient is moved into a 30-degree reverse Trendelenburg position, with the table rolled with the left side down to improve visualization of the critical structures and to bring the patient closer to the surgeon.
- The infundibulum of the gallbladder is pulled laterally by the surgeon's left hand when starting on the medial surface of the gallbladder. This distracts the cystic duct away from the common bile duct so that they are at right angles to each other. This will make identification of the cystic duct easier and helps to prevent inadvertent injury.
- The peritoneum overlying the lower edge of the gallbladder is opened using the hook electrocautery. The cystic node can be used to judge where the lower edge of the gallbladder is. The peritoneum overlying the node should be divided on the side abutting the gallbladder in order to avoid dividing the vessel coming up to the node. The node is then swept down, exposing the lower edge of the gallbladder (Figure 8-2).
- Once the peritoneum on the medial surface is divided, the gallbladder infundibulum is pulled medially, exposing the right side or "back side." Occasionally, a posterior branch of the artery is encountered as it branches off of the cystic artery below the gallbladder wall. It can be doubly clipped, or cauterized with the hook, and divided. Division of the peritoneum is continued all the way to the liver edge (Figure 8-3).
- The dissection should continue on the lower margin of the gallbladder. Identification of the wall and structures may require going back and forth, changing the position of the gallbladder and the angle of the 30-degree laparoscope, until the structures are defined.
- Every time the hook electrocautery is used, care should be taken to identify the tissue being divided. The inclination is to divide the deeper tissues, but this is not necessary until the peritoneum is divided on both sides. Being mindful to divide only "see-through" tissues will prevent the inadvertent division of vessels or ducts.
- The peanut or Maryland dissector is used for dissection of the hepatocystic triangle and stripping the structures to accommodate the clip applier.

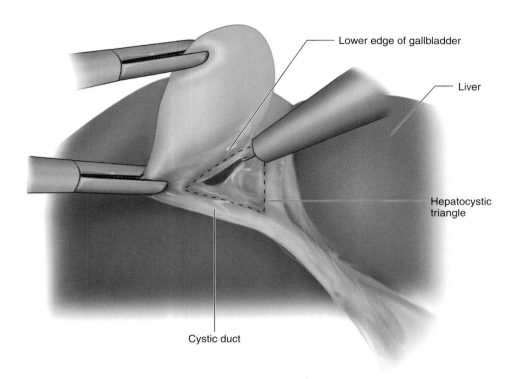

Lower edge of gallbladder

Liver

Hepatocystic triangle

Cystic duct

Figure 8-2

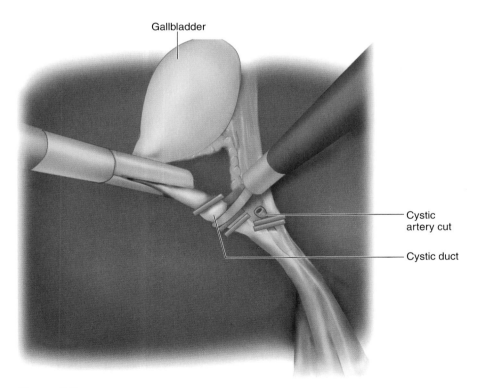

Gallbladder

Cystic artery cut

Cystic duct

Figure 8-3

- At this point, the gallbladder is removed from the liver bed using the "heel" of the hook instrument. Maintaining constant tension is critical to avoid entering the gallbladder or liver bed (Figure 8-4a and Figure 8-4b).
- If bleeding is encountered, control can be obtained by increasing the setting on the electrocautery. The instrument should be held above the surface of the liver to prevent the instrument from sticking to the liver and then dislodging the eschar. Begin cauterizing the most superior portions of the bleeding to avoid blood rolling down.
- Every effort should be made to extract stones when they spill in the abdomen. The stones can be picked up individually using stone forceps. To expedite this tedious task, the stones can be placed directly into a specimen retrieval bag within the abdomen. If there are many tiny fragments, then irrigant can be removed with a 10-mm suction device. Any bile spillage should be irrigated.
- The instruments and ports are removed from the abdomen as the CO_2 pneumoperitoneum is evacuated, and the skin is reapproximated.

Step 4. Postoperative Care

- Once liquids are tolerated and pain is controlled with oral medications, patients are able to leave the hospital. Most patients go home the same day the operation is performed.
- Patients can remove the dressings and shower the day after the operation.
- Activity depends on how the patient feels. Most patients will return to normal activities within a week.
- Patients are usually seen in the office 2 to 3 weeks after surgery.

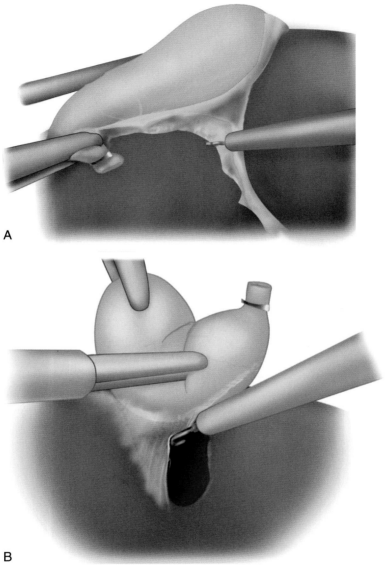

A

B

Figure 8-4

Step 5. Pearls and Pitfalls

- For patients who have had a prior midline incision or who have an umbilical defect, access is obtained using a Veress needle in the left upper quadrant, and the initial trocar is then placed in the lateral position.
- In obese patients whose umbilicus is displaced caudally, a port placed through the umbilicus will be too low for the surgeon to see the gallbladder clearly. Instead, the port is placed well above the umbilicus, usually around 20 cm below the xiphoid process.
- Very difficult procedures in which the patient is super morbidly obese can be made easier by performing the procedure using a split leg table with the surgeon operating from between the legs. The table is placed in a steep reverse Trendelenburg position to bring the operative field close to the surgeon.
- A very distended gallbladder can be decompressed with a laparoscopic needle aspirator so that the grasper used for retraction of the fundus is able to hold the tissue. When that instrument is unavailable, a Veress needle placed through the right upper quadrant abdominal wall can be introduced directly into the fundus and used to aspirate bile.
- Retrograde or "fundus-down technique" can be useful when a very inflamed gallbladder is encountered and the anatomy cannot be determined. The procedure is much like the standard open technique with dissection proceeding down along the gallbladder wall. The cystic duct can be transected at any safe level.
- If the liver is extremely large, there is excessive inflammation, or the gallbladder wall is not sturdy enough to be retracted, a liver retractor introduced through the right lateral port can hold the liver up and facilitate the dissection.

Selected Reference

Hunter JG: Avoidance of bile duct injury during laparoscopic cholecystectomy. *Am J Surgery* 162(1):71-76, 1991.
Way LW, Stewart LS, et al: Causes and prevention of laparoscopic bile duct injuries: analysis of 252 cases from a human factors and cognitive psychology perspective. *Annals of Surg* 237(4):460-9, 2003.

LIVER RESECTION (LEFT LATERAL SECTIONECTOMY)

Nicholas O'Rourke

Step 1. Surgical Anatomy

- Laparoscopic removal of the left lateral section of the liver can be very straightforward. For most surgeons, this will be their first "major" liver resection. However, there is still a real risk of disaster. Because of this combination of an easy procedure and intraoperative complications that are potentially life threatening, it is imperative that the surgeon understands the anatomy and instrumentation. Skill and experience with both open liver surgery and advanced laparoscopy remain essential.
- The left lateral section of the liver (formerly called the left lobe, now segments 2 and 3) is defined as the parenchyma to the left side of the falciform ligament. This ligament fans out over the surface of the left lateral section as Glissons capsule and condenses posteriorly as the left triangular ligament, attaching the liver to the undersurface of the diaphragm.
- The round ligament, or ligamentum teres, representing the usually obliterated umbilical vein, runs in the free edge of the falciform ligament, and enters the liver anterior to a variably thick bridge of liver tissue linking segments 3 and 4b. The caudate lobe lies posteriorly, separated from the left lateral section by the hepatogastric ligament or lesser omentum.
- The branching inflow to the left hemiliver lies just deep to the entry of the round ligament into the liver. Here the left portal triad of hepatic artery, bile duct, and portal vein divides with branching to segments 2 and 3 on the left and segment 4 on the right.
- The left lateral section is drained by the left hepatic vein, which usually joins with the middle vein before entering the vena cava. The left vein has a variable extrahepatic course, but its left side can be exposed by mobilizing the left lateral section.

Step 2. Preoperative Considerations

Patient Preparation

- Liver resection should always be undertaken for a valid reason, whether open or laparoscopic.
- Tumors are removed because of known malignancy, uncertain diagnosis, or symptoms.
- Tumors must lie well clear of the line of transection (i.e., the line of the falciform ligament).

- Good preoperative imaging with multiphase computed tomography (CT) or magnetic resonance imaging (MRI) is essential. This is the one liver operation where intraoperative ultrasound is not always essential, because of the clear sectional definition by the falciform ligament.
- Resection will be much easier in a healthy, slim, nonsteatotic liver.
- Enlarged fatty livers can be greatly improved by placing the patient on a high-protein, very low calorie diet for 2 weeks.
- The surgeon must understand the principles of open liver surgery and have skills in advanced laparoscopic surgery, such as suturing.

Equipment and Instrumentation

- Reusable and disposable instruments
- Specialized equipment (i.e., staplers, clip appliers, balloon ports)
- Cautery and devices for hemostasis

Anesthesia

- Antibiotics
- NGT Nasogastric tube (NGT), Foley catheter, Foley

Room Setup and Patient Positioning

- The patient is supine and under general anesthetic.
- The surgeon stands on the right side of the patient with the monitor over the patient's head or left shoulder (Figure 9-1).

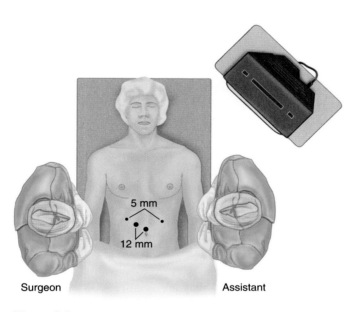

5 mm

12 mm

Surgeon

Assistant

Figure 9-1

Step 3. Operative Steps

Access and Port Placement

- Access is via the umbilicus with a 12-mm Hassan canula, or elsewhere in the upper abdomen if adhesions are expected. Carbon dioxide is insufflated to the lowest pressure permitting visualization (because of risk of embolization).
- Two to three working ports are needed. One of these needs to be a 12 mm size for linear stapler access. With experience, only two 5-mm ports are needed and a 5-mm, 30-degree laparoscope is used. It is best if the large port traverses the umbilicus.
- The left lateral section is mobilized by dividing the left triangular ligament, watching for the gastroesophageal junction posteriorly and the pericardium anteriorly. The left phrenic vein will be seen entering the left hepatic vein (Figure 9-2).
- The bridge of liver tissue overlying the round ligament is divided, and the left lateral section is lifted by placing a grasper or sucker beneath and medial, to feel the potential vascular control that can be achieved by such a maneuver.
- The round ligament can be preserved or divided to allow best access to the line of transection, usually just to the left of the falciform ligament (Figure 9-3).
- Liver transection can be performed with a variety of instruments, just as in open surgery. The simplest and quickest technique is to use a linear cutting stapler such as the Endo-GIA (Covidien, Mansfield, Massachusetts). My preference is for a 60-mm vascular (2.0 white) load with articulation.
- Correct stapler technique means taking the liver in layers in almost all instances. Two or three layers of staple firings are needed, using up to nine loads. The trick is to take no more than 15 mm of liver thickness in one bite, with the thin arm of the stapler gently insinuated into the liver substance until resistance (usually a vessel) is felt.

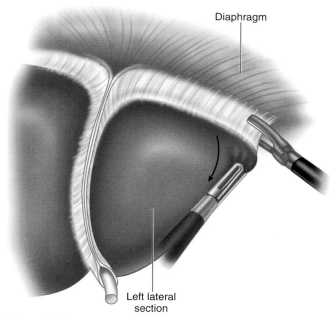

Diaphragm

Left lateral
section

Figure 9-2

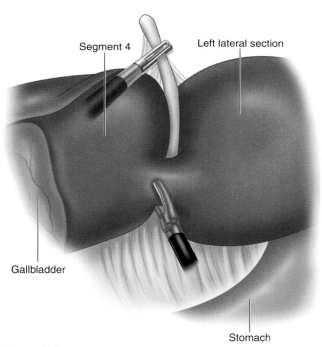

Segment 4   Left lateral section

Gallbladder

Stomach

Figure 9-3

- If the patient is very slim, as may be the case in thin females, then it may be possible to take the whole left lateral section in two or three firings. Glisson's capsule pinches down on itself giving a reassuring hemostatic seal (Figure 9-4).
- Particularly on the less vascular anterior half of the resection, other devices, such as laparoscopic bipolar shears, Ligasure (Covidien, Mansfield, Massachusetts), or ultrasonic coagulating shears, Harmonic (Ethicon, Somerville, New Jersey) shears, can be used.
- When using the LigaSure, first you crush the parenchyma as with "Kelly clysis" in open liver surgery. Best results will be achieved with the power on as the jaws close, using copious irrigation to prevent sticking and not firing the blade until the crushed tissue is observed. With this technique, intact vessels will be seen and can be burned, clipped, or stapled. LigaSure is now preferred, as, if used correctly, vessels will be preserved, rather than harmonic shears, which will divide vessels.
- Any bleeding can usually be controlled by the lifting up maneuver, with an instrument placed in the groove of the hepatogastric ligament and pressed up and to the right (Figure 9-5) or with direct pressure over the bleeder. Completion of the resection with staplers may stop hemorrhage, but occasionally, suturing is required.
- Laparoscopic control is preferred to conversion, but if progress is slow, conversion is essential.
- The cut surface is then inspected for bile leaks, which can be clipped or sutured.
- The specimen can be removed whole through a lower abdominal incision. If benign, then it can be morcellated and taken out via the umbilicus.

Step 4. Postoperative Care

- Drains are rarely needed.
- Recovery should be similar to that following laparoscopic cholecystectomy.
- Most patients are home within 24 hours.
- As in all types of laparoscopic surgery, be aware that symptoms beyond 48 hours may reflect a complication.

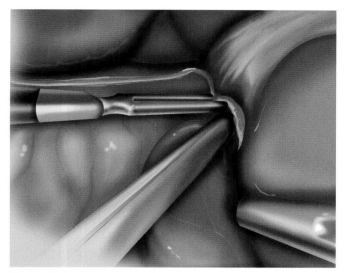

Figure 9-4

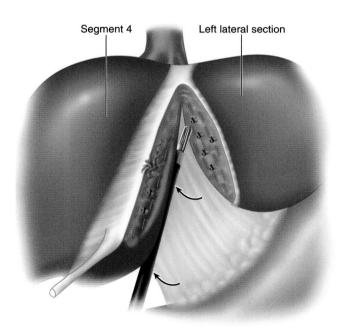

Figure 9-5

Step 5. Pearls and Pitfalls

- This is the easiest of liver resections, open or laparoscopic.
- Patients can still die, from bleeding, or injury to adjacent organs, such as the heart or esophagus.
- Do not use staplers for the first time on a vascular organ in a live human. Become familiar with them first. They must be kept rock steady when firing, as slight movements of the surgeon's hand can be magnified and lead to tearing of vessels. Make certain that the position of both blades is known before firing, as once used, there is no going back!
- Carbon dioxide gas embolism is not a clinical problem. Air embolism can be. Argon embolization from argon beam coagulation devices has been reported and if using, one must open a port to vent the abdomen and never apply the beam over an open vein.

Selected References

Chang S, Laurent A, Tayar C, et al: Laparoscopy as a routine approach for left lateral sectionectomy. *Brit J Surg* 94(1):58-63, 2007.
O'Rourke N, Shaw I, Nathanson L, et al: Laparoscopic resection of hepatic colorectal metastases. HPB, 6(4):230-35, 2004.
Strasberg S, Pang YY: The Brisbane 2000 terminology of liver anatomy and resections, IHPBA. HPB, vol 2, 333-339, 2000.

Solid Organ Surgery

10

TRANSGASTRIC CYSTGASTROSTOMY

Douglas S. Smink

Step 1. Surgical Anatomy

- Preoperative imaging, typically an abdominal computed tomography scan, is imperative to determine the location of the pancreatic pseudocyst relative to the stomach. For the transgastric approach, the cyst needs to be directly posterior to the stomach.
- Attention should be paid to the location of the splenic artery, to make certain that it is not at risk for injury when creating the cystgastrostomy.
- If the cyst is not directly posterior to the stomach, an alternative approach is necessary. A cystojejunostomy is ideal in such cases and can often be performed laparoscopically.

Step 2. Preoperative Considerations

Patient Preparation

- The diagnosis of pancreatic pseudocyst should be firmly established. The patient typically has a history of pancreatitis, but further investigation is necessary to confirm the diagnosis.
- Preoperative evaluation includes a computed tomography scan to determine the size and location of the cyst, as well as an endoscopic retrograde cholangiopancreatogram (ERCP) to assess for communication between the pancreatic duct and the cyst.
- In some instances, endoscopic ultrasound or aspiration of the cyst for amylase and lipase levels may be warranted. Pancreatic pseudocysts typically have high levels of amylase and lipase.
- Once the diagnosis of pseudocyst is made, the cyst wall should be allowed to mature for at least 6 weeks prior to surgical drainage.

Equipment and Instrumentation

♦ The following equipment is needed: a 5-mm, 30-degree laparoscope, a flexible upper endoscope, a percutaneous endoscopic gastrostomy (PEG) kit, balloon or buttressed 5-mm ports, a gallbladder aspirator, ultrasonic sheers, and an endoscopic ultrasound (if available).

Anesthesia

♦ After the induction of general anesthesia, a Foley catheter should be placed and a first-generation cephalosporin should be administered.
♦ An orogastric tube is not necessary, as the procedure begins with an endoscopy.

Patient Positioning

♦ The patient is placed supine on the operating room table in the split-leg position with the arms tucked at the sides.

Step 3. Operative Steps

Percutaneous Endoscopic Gastrostomy Tube Placement

♦ A percutaneous endoscopic gastrostomy (PEG) tube is placed in standard fashion. This creates apposition of the anterior gastric wall to the anterior abdominal wall.

Port Placement

♦ A 5-mm trocar is placed through the PEG tube to allow insufflation of the stomach with carbon dioxide to 15 mm Hg. Two additional 5-mm trocars are placed on either side of the PEG. The endoscope is used to visualize placement of these trocars. Following placement of the trocars, the endoscope is retracted back into the midesophagus. Ideally, the additional trocars should have an internal buttress or balloon to ensure apposition of the anterior gastric wall to the anterior abdominal wall (Figure 10-1).

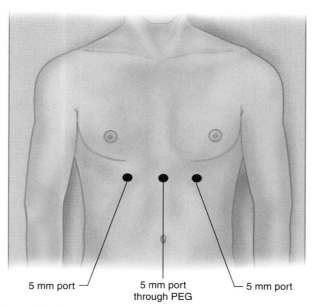

5 mm port ────   5 mm port   ──── 5 mm port
                                  through PEG

Figure 10-1

- Alternatively, no PEG is placed, and the trocars are inserted directly into the gastric lumen with laparoscopic guidance. In this technique, intraperitoneal access is obtained at the umbilicus, and the peritoneum is insufflated to 5 to 8 mm Hg. An endoscope is passed into the stomach, and the stomach is insufflated. Three balloon trocars are then inserted through the upper abdomen and into the gastric lumen. The balloons are then inflated, and the gastric wall is pulled against the abdominal wall. The stomach is then insufflated while the peritoneum is desufflated.

Cyst Localization

- The cyst is localized with an aspirator. In most instances, the cyst makes a visible bulge in the posterior stomach (Figure 10-2).
- If the location of the cyst is not obvious, intraoperative ultrasound can be used. After aspiration of the cyst confirms cyst fluid, the aspirator is left in place in the posterior gastric wall.

Creation of Cystgastrostomy

- With the aspirator still in place to confirm the location of the cyst, a cystgastrostomy is created with the ultrasonic shears adjacent to the aspirator. The aspirator is then withdrawn, and the cystgastrostomy is enlarged with the ultrasonic shears (Figure 10-3). Alternatively, the laparoscopic stapler may be used in the patient when there is bleeding at the cystogastrostomy or if the area seems particularly well-vascularized.
- A portion of the cyst wall should be sent for pathologic evaluation. Hook cautery can also be used to expand the opening.
- Suction should be available to remove the liquid contents of the cyst.
- Bleeding is typically minimal. If bleeding persists from the edge of the cystgastrostomy, it can be controlled with sutures.

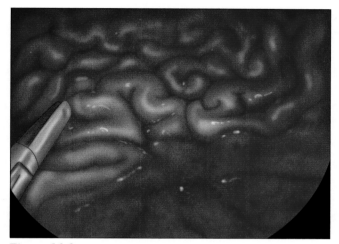

Figure 10-2

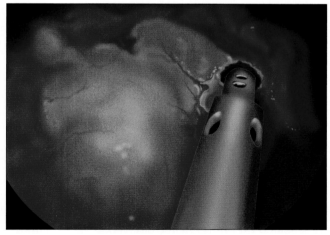

Figure 10-3

Endoscopy of the Cyst

◆ To ensure adequate drainage of the cyst, the endoscope is again passed into the stomach, through the cystgastrostomy, and into the pseudocyst. The cystgastrostomy should be large enough (approximately 2 cm) to permit passage of a standard endoscope. Any remaining cyst contents can be aspirated through the endoscope (Figure 10-4).

Removal of Trocars and Closure of Gastrotomies

◆ The stomach is desufflated and the endoscope is removed. The trocars are backed out of the stomach such that they now only traverse the abdominal wall. The PEG is removed as well, and a new trocar is placed through the abdominal wall where the PEG had been. The abdomen is now insufflated, creating a typical laparoscopic environment.
◆ The three anterior gastrotomies are sutured closed laparoscopically. In some instances, a fourth 5-mm trocar is inserted to provide optimal suturing of the anterior gastric wall (Figure 10-5).
◆ The abdomen is then desufflated, all trocars are removed, and the skin incisions are closed.

Step 4. Postoperative Care

◆ The patient is placed on clear liquids postoperatively and admitted for observation overnight. Regular diet can be initiated on postoperative day 1 and the patient discharged home later that day.

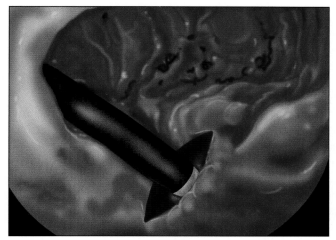

Figure 10-4

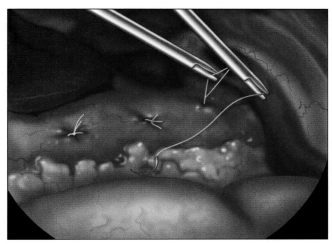

Figure 10-5

Step 5. Pearls and Pitfalls

- The pseudocyst should be localized directly posterior to the posterior wall of the stomach to enable this approach.
- A large PEG tube should be used to enable passage of a 5-mm trocar.
- The cystgastrostomy should be sufficiently large (approximately 2 cm in diameter) to allow adequate drainage of the pseudocyst.
- This approach makes it difficult to adequately biopsy the cyst wall. If the diagnosis of pseudocyst is not certain and there is concern for malignancy, an alternative approach that enables a biopsy should be performed. A laparoscopic stapled cystgastrostomy is an excellent alternative in this instance.

Selected References

Bergmann S, Melvin WS: Operative and nonoperative management of pancreatic pseudocysts. *Surg Clin N Am* 87(6):1447-60, 2007.
Mori T, Abe N, Sugiyama M, et al: Laparoscopic pancreatic cystgastrostomy. *J Hepatobiliary Pancreat Surg* 7(1):28-34, 2000.

11

DISTAL PANCREATIC RESECTION

Thai H. Pham, Erin W. Gilbert, Swee H. Teh, and Brett C. Sheppard

Step 1. Surgical Anatomy

- The most common indications for performing distal pancreatectomy are benign or malignant neoplasm, complications of pancreatitis, and occasionally trauma.
- Although there has been extensive literature on the role of open distal pancreatectomy for malignant disease, there is only a nascent literature on the role of laparoscopic distal pancreatectomy.
- Laparoscopic distal pancreatectomy remains a procedure usually conducted for benign pancreatic disease. This chapter reviews the perioperative care and discusses the operative techniques for laparoscopic distal pancreatectomy.

Step 2. Preoperative Consideration

Patient Preparation

- A contrast-enhanced computed tomography (CT) scan utilizing a pancreatic protocol is obtained for preoperative assessment of pancreatic disease. This study provides images of the pancreas during arterial and venous phases to allow for a full evaluation of smaller lesions and to help delineate the relationship of the splenic vessels to the lesion.
- Patients with radiographic abnormalities of the body and tail of the pancreas usually undergo endoscopic ultrasound with or without FNA (fine needle aspiration) and cystic fluid sampling if indicated.
- In patients with a dilated pancreatic duct, an Endoscopic Retrograde Cholangiopancreatography (ERCP) may be useful for evaluating the papilla and ductal anatomy and its relationship to the lesion. Alternatively, Magnetic Resonance Cholangiopancreatography (MRCP) is also useful as a noninvasive means for elucidating pancreatic pathology and anatomy.
- In our institution, a pancreas protocol CT and EUS (Endoscopic Ultrasound) fully assess the majority of patients and obviate the need for additional studies.

- If splenectomy is anticipated, then preoperative vaccination against encapsulated bacteria (H. Influenza, Streptococcus, Meningococcus) should be given 7 to 10 days before surgery.
- Patients with functional pancreatic neuroendocrine tumors may require preoperative hospitalization to optimize physiologic status.
- Similar to other major abdominal surgeries, preoperative antibiotics and DVT (deep venous thrombosis) prophylaxis are provided per Surgical Care Improvement Project (SCIP) guidelines.

Equipment and Instrumentation

- For a laparoscopic approach, a 30-degree and 45-degree laparoscope, ultrasonic dissector, 5-mm and 10-mm clip applier, blunt-tipped atraumatic bowel graspers, fine-tipped needle driver, articulating endoscopic stapler, fibrin glue with laparoscopic delivery device, and hand port should be available.
- In addition, a laparoscopic ultrasound should be available to help locate and characterize lesions intraoperatively. The ultrasound is often particularly useful for clarifying the spatial relationship of neuroendocrine tumors to the main pancreatic duct. In addition, intraoperative ultrasound may help explain other occult pathology, which may change intraoperative decision-making.

Anesthesia

- General anesthesia with endotracheal intubation and complete neuromuscular blockade is generally required for this operation.
- After intubation, a nasogastric (NG) tube should be placed to decompress the stomach during the operation and for patient care during the immediate postoperative period.
- A Foley catheter should be placed and standard preoperative antibiotics given per surgeon.

Room Setup and Patient Positioning

♦ The patient is positioned in a 30-degree right lateral decubitus position using a beanbag or large gel rolls. This allows for rotation of the patient during mobilization of the pancreas and allows the use of gravity as a retractor during the case. The 30-degree lateral decubitus also provides for rotation into a horizontal position if conversion to an open procedure is required.
  ▲ The left arm will often need to be placed in a padded cradle "airplane" position and gently fixed out of the operative field. The upper and lower extremities are well padded, and the patient is carefully secured to the table.
  ▲ This procedure can also be done with the patient in supine position. The surgeon stands between the patient's legs and the assistant stands to the left of the patient. This position is best for medial-to-lateral dissection.

Step 3. Operative Steps

♦ There are several technical variations that may be utilized based on surgeon preference and characteristics of the operative field.
♦ Pancreatic mobilization can be performed from lateral to medial or from medial to lateral. In general, the lateral-to-medial approach is often easier. However, this does not allow for early control of the splenic artery and vein.
♦ For extended distal pancreatic resections, we often prefer to proceed from medial to lateral, beginning with division of the neck of the pancreas. This facilitates later dissection by allowing early control of the splenic vessels. The medial-to-lateral approach is also useful to aid mobilization of the vessels when splenic preservation is considered. Complete splenic mobilization is not necessary unless the spleen is to be removed.
♦ We will describe laparoscopic distal pancreatectomy with en bloc splenectomy via a medial-to-lateral approach and follow this with a discussion of how splenic preservation can be done laparoscopically.

Access and Port Placement

- Pneumoperitoneum is achieved by either the Veress needle technique, with the needle placed through the umbilicus, or the open Hassan technique at the site of the operating laparoscope. The laparoscopic distal pancreatic resection is performed via four trocars.
- A critical component of any laparoscopic approach is port placement.
- The locations of these trocars may vary slightly depending on the body habitus of the patient. In general, the trocars should be triangulated around the body and tail of the pancreas with a working distance that allows sufficient range of motion.
- We have obtained the greatest flexibility by utilizing three 12-mm trocars and one 5-mm trocar.
- Figure 11-1 outlines the position of the trocars. In general, a 12-mm trocar is placed in the supraumbilical position to the left of the midline, and exploratory laparoscopy is performed. A 12-mm trocar is placed just 5 cm lateral to the left midclavicular line. This trocar will allow passage of the flexible laparoscopic ultrasound probe and the articulated endoscopic staple device. The assistant's port is a 5-mm trocar placed in the left midclavicular line approximately 10 cm above the camera port. If necessary this position can be converted into a hand port during the operation. Finally, a fourth 12-mm trocar is placed in the right midclavicular line approximately 5 cm above the camera port. An additional 5-mm subxiphoid trocar can be added, retracting the left lobe of the liver if necessary.
- In general, the principles of laparoscopic resection are similar to an open distal pancreatectomy.

Lesser Sac Exposure

- To access the lesser sac, the patient is first placed in a reverse Trendelenburg position to allow gravity to drop the great omentum and the small bowel from the operating field. If a large left lobe of the liver obscures the stomach, a Nathanson or other liver retractor should be placed in the epigastrium and the left lobe retracted.
- The assistant retracts the stomach in an anterior and cephalad direction. Using an ultrasonic dissector, the lesser sac is entered by dividing the gastrocolic omentum along the greater curvature of the stomach, with care to avoid injury to the right gastroepiploic vessels. This dissection can usually be started 5 cm proximal to the pylorus on the greater curve of the stomach. Care must be taken to avoid contact with the gastric wall to prevent thermal injury from the ultrasonic dissector.

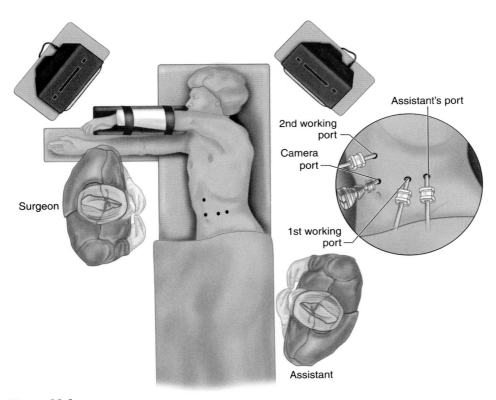

Surgeon

2nd working port

Assistant's port

Camera port

1st working port

Assistant

Figure 11-1

- Alternatively, the lesser sac can be entered through the avascular plane superior to the transverse colon, but this option may leave the greater omentum in the operative field. The mobilization is continued proximally along the greater curvature by dividing all of the short gastric vessels. Congenital adhesions between the posterior wall of the stomach and the pancreas are divided, and the lesser sac is fully visualized.
- In patients with chronic pancreatitis or desmoplastic reaction from a pancreatic neuroendocrine tumor, there may be significant adhesions in this lesser sac space, and careful dissection to mobilize the posterior wall of the stomach will be necessary. To maintain exposure of the pancreas within the lesser sac, the stomach is secured to the anterior abdominal wall using percutaneously inserted T fasteners or laparoscopically placed sutures.
- Once the pancreatic body and tail are exposed, laparoscopic ultrasound can assist in locating and determining morphology and respectability of the pancreatic lesion.

Splenic Flexure Mobilization

- The splenocolic attachments are divided with the ultrasonic dissector to further expose the inferior pole of the spleen and pancreatic tail. Depending on the patient's anatomy, the left colon may be in the way and will need to be mobilized by dividing its retroperitoneal attachments along the white line of Toldt. Although not always necessary, the mobilization and retraction of the left colon medially may provide greater exposure of the inferior pancreatic grove in order to develop a posterior retroperitoneal plane needed during mobilization of the pancreas.
- The splenic attachments to the diaphragm are not divided. These attachments will provide lateral retraction to prevent the spleen from entering the operative field during extremes of patient positioning (Figure 11-2).

Pancreatic Mobilization with Splenectomy

- Pancreatic mobilization begins by dividing the retroperitoneal attachments medial along the inferior pancreatic groove just proximal to the lesion. This allows for the development of an avascular retroperitoneal plane posterior to the pancreas, which can be extended cephalad and laterally. This retroperitoneal dissection plane can be difficult to identify, especially with senescent pancreas, and gentle probing will aid in identifying the transition point from firm pancreas to loose fatty areolar tissue in the inferior pancreatic grove. As this dissection plane is developed in the cephalad direction, the splenic vessels will be encountered. The cephalad dissection is complete if the posterior gastric wall can be seen with elevation of the pancreas.
- The dissection continues laterally toward the tail of the pancreas. Loose areolar tissue in this plane can be divided with the ultrasonic dissector. Care must be taken to maintain a horizontal plane of dissection, as the retropancreatic space is developed to avoid injuring retroperitoneal structures such as the kidney and adrenal gland. This is usually a significant issue in the operative field when there has been extensive preoperative inflammation.

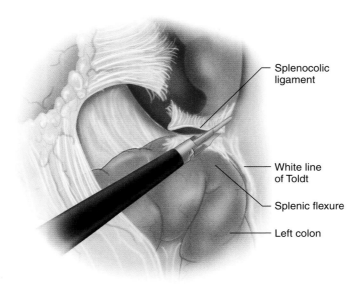

Splenocolic
ligament

White line
of Toldt

Splenic flexure

Left colon

Figure 11-2

- If splenic preservation is to be performed, the splenic vein must be mobilized from its posterior-inferior position nestled along the pancreas. There will be numerous small venous tributaries draining into the splenic vein. Having a vessel loop around the vein will facilitate finding and dissecting these small veins. These small vessels are best divided with ultrasonic dissector, or they can be clipped with a 5-mm clip applier.

Mobilization of the Pancreas in the Retropancreatic Plane

- As the splenic vein and artery are encountered during the posterior pancreatic mobilization, they should be circumferentially dissected and controlled with vessel loops. Control of these two vessels should be done proximal to the pancreatic lesion and is critical if splenic vessel preservation is considered. By having control of these vessels, hemostasis can be achieved if bleeding is encountered during distal dissection.
- Splenic vessel dissection can be facilitated with a right angle dissector. Care should be taken to avoid injury to the left adrenal gland, which can be intimately associated with the tail of the pancreas and cause troublesome bleeding that will make further laparoscopic dissection difficult.

Pancreatic Transection: Parenchyma, Splenic Artery, and Vein

- It is preferable to isolate and separately divide the splenic artery, vein, and pancreatic parenchyma. Isolation of the splenic artery can be achieved at the superior border of the pancreas using a laparoscopic right angle dissector and ultrasonic dissector. In some instances, the splenic artery is more accessible through the posterior pancreatic dissection plane. At least 1.5 cm of exposed vessel is needed for the application of an articulating 30- to 45-mm endoscopic stapler. Alternatively, endoclips and scissors can be used if the vessels are of smaller caliber. An Endoloop can be applied to the proximal stump of the artery to reinforce the endoclips. The splenic vein can also be stapled with an endoscopic 45-mm vascular stapler (Figure 11-3).
- Pancreas transection can be performed with either an endoscopic vascular stapler if the pancreas is soft or a reticulating Endo GIA stapler (Covidien, Mansfield, Massachusetts) if the pancreas is thick or firm. Care must be taken to visualize the tip of the stapler prior to firing to ensure clearance of other surrounding structures including other branches of the celiac axis. Gentle and slow firing of the stapler may improve hemostasis and prevent unnecessary traumatic injury to the pancreas.
- The spleen is then freed of its attachments to the diaphragm and retroperitoneum, and the specimen is ready for extraction.

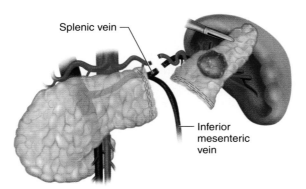

Figure 11-3

Pancreatic Stump Management

◆ The main pancreatic duct is not routinely identified within the stapled end of the pancreas. The entire end of the gland is oversewn in a running or mattressed fashion using 3-0 Prolene suture. The resection bed is then irrigated and inspected for hemostasis. The stapled splenic artery and vein ends are reinspected. The oversewn pancreatic stump is then covered with tissue sealant using a laparoscopic delivery system.

Splenic Preserving Distal Pancreatic Resection

◆ There are two methods of spleen preservation during the laparoscopic distal pancreatic resection. The first preserves the splenic artery and vein, therefore maintaining the inflow and outflow of the spleen. The second method, described by Warshaw, ligates these vessels while preserving the short gastric vessels. This method has been questioned because of a potentially higher risk of splenic infarct and the development of gastric varices (Figure 11-4).
◆ It has been demonstrated that splenic artery and vein preservation is necessary to maintain the immunologic function of the spleen. Therefore, it is our preference to preserve the splenic artery and vein with careful dissection (Figure 11-5).

Specimen Removal

◆ The distal pancreas and spleen can be removed using an Endo Catch bag through a 12-mm port. The spleen can be morcellated in the Endo Catch bag to avoid having to enlarge the fascial defect at the port site. However, we find parsimonious extension of the fascial defect facilitates specimen delivery, omits the need for splenic morcellation, and does not contribute significantly to incisional morbidity or convalescence.
◆ If the procedure was done for pancreatic neoplasm, the proximal pancreatic stump of the specimen should be marked and sent for frozen section analysis by pathology. Pathologic confirmation of any potential neuroendocrine lesion also needs to be accomplished.

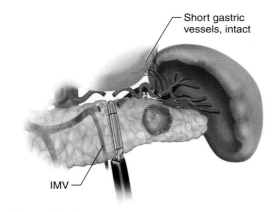

Figure 11-4

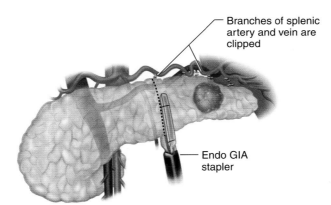

Figure 11-5

Drain Placement and Closure

- The resection bed is irrigated and hemostasis is checked, and a closed suction drain is inserted near the pancreatic bed and brought out through the 5-mm trocar site. The pneumoperitoneum is released and all trocars are removed under direct vision. Fascial incisions greater than 10 mm should be closed.

Step 4. Postoperative Care

- The patient can be typically cared for on the regular surgical ward with intravenous fluids and pain medications.
- The NG tube can be removed the following day and clear liquids can be initiated as tolerated.
- Patients are encouraged to ambulate and use incentive spirometry as early as possible to prevent DVT and atelectasis.
- In the absence of a large wound, perioperative morbidities including wound infections, ileus, and cardiopulmonary compromise remain less than 20%. The overall perioperative mortality is less than 1%.
- Pancreatic leak remains a challenging problem in the laparoscopic approach as in the open. A surgical drain is left in place until the patient is tolerating regular diet and drain output is less than 30 mL per day. Drain fluid is not routinely sent for analysis unless there is concern for pancreatic stump leak, which can be indicated by high volume output, persistent intra-abdominal irritation manifested most commonly by fever, ileus, or lack of clinical improvement. Most leaks will stop with conservative treatment.
- Uncomplicated hospitalizations typically range from 3 to 5 days.

Step 5. Pearls and Pitfalls

- There are several pitfalls to consider while mobilizing the medial pancreas. The inferior mesenteric vein (IMV) is often located just lateral to the ligament of Treitz in the retroperitoneum at the midportion of the body of the pancreas. Attempts to save the IMV as it courses superiorly to join the splenic vein should be made to decrease the risk of splenic and portal vein thrombosis (see Figure 11-4).
- Dissection and control of the splenic vessels is described, where the vessels are controlled as they are encountered during posterior mobilization of the pancreas. This approach is useful for dissecting the splenic vein, but it may be more difficult for dissecting the splenic artery, depending on patient's anatomy. If this is the case, the *splenic artery can be mobilized* and controlled first by dissecting along the superior pancreatic edge (see Figure 11-3).
- The dissection of the splenic vein is challenging because of its thin wall and numerous branches. The venous branches can usually be divided with an ultrasonic dissector without much bleeding. The one exception here is when varices are encountered. To assure optimal hemostasis, *varices* must be divided by the use of endoclips and not an ultrasonic dissector. If endoclips are used to control vascular branches, then care should be taken to make sure that they do not prevent the proper firing of the endoscopic stapler when dividing the main vessels.
- If the dissection of the vessels is difficult because of the inability to attain adequate exposure, then a *hand port* may be placed to facilitate exposure.

Selected References

Fernandez-Cruz L, Orduna D, Cesar-Borges G, et al: Distal pancreatectomy: en-bloc splenectomy vs spleen-preserving pancreatectomy. *HPB* 7(2):93-98, 2005.

Kooby DA, Gillespie T, Bentrem D, et al: Left-sided pancreatectomy: a multicenter comparison of laparoscopic and open approaches. *Ann Surg* 248(3):438-46, 2008.

Leemans R, Manson W, Snijder JA, et al: Immune response capacity after human splenic autotransplantation: restoration of response to individual pneumococcal vaccine subtypes. *Ann Surg* 229(2):279-85, 1999.

Pryor A, Means JR, Pappas TN: Laparoscopic distal pancreatectomy with splenic preservation. *Surg Endosc* 21(12):2326-30, 2007.

Warshaw AL: Conservation of the spleen with distal pancreatectomy. *Arch Surg* 123(5):550-53, 1988.

Teh SH, Tseng D, Sheppard BC: Laparoscopic and open distal pancreatic resection for benign pancreatic disease. *J Gastrointest Surg* 11(9):1120-25, 2007.

CHAPTER 12

PANCREATICOJEJUNOSTOMY (PUESTOW PROCEDURE)

Ali Tavakkolizadeh

Step 1. Surgical Anatomy

- The exocrine pancreas is drained via a main and an accessory duct (Figure 12-1).
- The main pancreatic duct is often affected in chronic pancreatitis. Preoperative ERCP (Endoscopic Retrograde Cholangiopancreatography) is effective in demonstrating ductal dilatation and the presence of stones (Figure 12-2).

Step 2. Preoperative Considerations

Patient Preparation

- To be considered for this procedure, patients must have failed conservative medical therapy and be managed by a multidisciplinary team, including primary care and gastroenterology.
- Patients should undergo appropriate pre-operative imaging, including a high-resolution computed tomography (CT) and ERCP, or Magnetic Resonance Cholangiopancreatography (MRCP) (Figure 12-2).
- It is critical to assess pancreatic duct dilatation and ductal strictures, and to rule out the presence of a potentially malignant mass.
- The pancreatic duct should be dilated to greater than 7 mm in diameter.
- Preoperative placement of a pancreatic stent for temporary pain relief may be appropriate. This is not a contraindication to surgery.
- Many patients will have nutritional deficiencies and diabetes. Appropriate treatment should be initiated for these comorbidities before these patients undergo surgery.
- Informed consent should be obtained. It is important to set expectations appropriately. The patients should not expect cure, but a 70% to 80% improvement in pain.

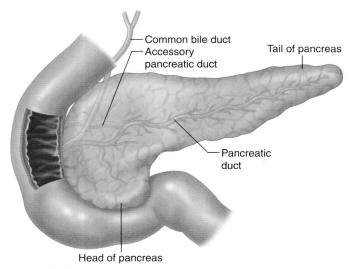

Figure 12-1

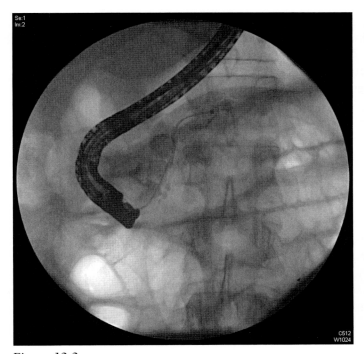

Figure 12-2

Equipment and Instrumentation

- Disposable laparoscopic ports
- 30-degree, 10-mm laparoscope
- Endoscopic staplers
- Laparoscopic suturing instruments (EndoStitch)
- Harmonic scalpel for hemostasis
- Laparoscopic needle aspirator and laparoscopic ultrasound to help identify the pancreatic duct

Anesthesia

General anesthesia is given and the following interventions done during this stage:
- Administration of preoperative antibiotics (e.g., Ancef) 1 hour prior to the skin incision
- Subcutaneous heparin
- Nasogastric tube placement
- Foley catheter placement

Room Setup and Patient Positioning

- The patient is placed in split-leg position, and foot plates are used to prevent sliding.
- Monitors are placed above the patient's head.
- The operative surgeon usually stands on the patient's right side with the assistant at the patient's left side. The surgeon may find it helpful to move to the position between the legs during certain parts of the procedure (e.g., dissection of the pancreas medially).

Step 3. Operative Steps

Access and Port Placement

- A Veress needle is introduced along the left subcostal margin, in the midclavicular line, and a pneumoperitoneum is created to a pressure of 15 mmHg using carbon dioxide.
- A 12-mm camera port is placed 3 cm to the left of midline and approximately 8 cm above the umbilicus. A 10-mm, 30-degree laparoscope is then introduced into the peritoneal space.
- Under direct vision, a 12-mm working port is placed 4 cm to the right of the midline and 6 to 8 cm above the umbilicus. A 5-mm working port is placed in the right upper quadrant. An assistant 5-mm port is placed in the left upper quadrant.
- A 5-mm incision is made in the subxiphoid space, and the Nathanson retractor is introduced to elevate the left lobe of the liver.

Exposing the Lesser Sac

- Using the Harmonic scalpel, the gastrocolic ligament is divided below the gastroepiploic vessels and the lesser sac is entered.
- The greater curve is mobilized from the pylorus to the fundus to provide adequate exposure of the lesser sac and the pancreas. There are often inflammatory attachments between the posterior gastric wall and the pancreas, which need to be divided.
- The Nathanson retractor is then gently repositioned to elevate the stomach and maintain exposure of the lesser sac.

Identification of the Pancreas and Pancreatic Duct

◆ The peritoneum along the superior and inferior border of the pancreas is divided and the pancreas clearly identified and exposed (Figure 12-3).
◆ The splenic vessels are visualized and preserved.
◆ The pancreatic head, neck, and body are typically thickened and fibrotic, with some distortion of the normal anatomy.
◆ The pancreatic duct is identified by inserting a laparoscopic needle aspirator in the pancreatic parenchyma, where the duct is thought to be situated (Figure 12-4).
◆ When available, an intraoperative ultrasound can assist with this.
◆ Aspiration of pancreatic fluid confirms the duct position.
◆ In patients with a preoperative pancreatic stent in place, duct identification can be easier.

Opening of the Pancreatic Duct and Stone Extraction

◆ Using electrocautery, the pancreatic duct is entered in the body and opened longitudinally for the entire length of the pancreas, starting 1 to 2 cm away from the duodenal border and going distally, as far as possible. The ductotomy should be at least 7 cm in length.
◆ The duct should be thoroughly examined and all stones removed. A review of the preoperative imaging can be helpful for identifying the relative position of the stones; these ductal regions should be carefully evaluated (Figure 12-5).

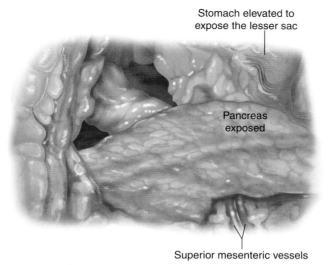

Figure 12-3

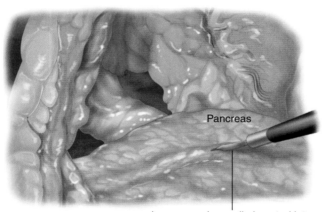

Figure 12-4

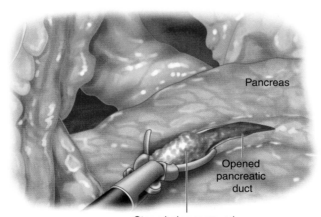

Figure 12-5

Creation of the Roux Limb

- The transverse colon is elevated to identify the ligament of Treitz.
- The jejunum is divided 40 cm distal to the ligament of Treitz using an endoscopic stapler (e.g., Endo-GIA 2.5 × 60 mm stapler, Covidien, Mansfield, Massachusetts). The mesentery of the small bowel is divided with the Harmonic device.
- A 50-cm Roux limb is measured and a side-to-side stapled jejunojejunostomy is created. To do this, the loops of bowel are approximated using an interrupted 2-0 silk suture. Enterotomies are made in the opposing segments of the small bowel using a Harmonic scalpel or hook electrocautery. A side-to-side jejunojejunostomy is created by two firings of the Endo-GIA 2.5 × 60 mm stapler in opposing directions. The common enterotomy is closed using another firing of the 2.5 × 60 mm Endo-GIA stapler. The mesenteric defect is closed using a running 2-0 silk suture (Figure 12-6).
- An opening is made in the transverse mesocolon, through the avascular area above the ligament of Treitz. The Roux limb is passed in a retrocolic fashion and placed over the pancreas. This should have no tension.

Pancreaticojejunostomy

- A laparoscopic one-layered pancreaticojejunostomy is performed. The distal end of Roux limb is sutured using an interrupted 2-0 silk suture to the pancreatic parenchyma at the tail of the pancreas. The small bowel is opened for the same length as the pancreatic duct has been exposed.
- A 2-0 Vicryl suture is used as a running suture, to create a pancreaticojejunostomy, starting at the tail of the pancreas and moving toward the midline, taking full bites of the bowel wall and the pancreatic duct (Figure 12-7).
- A second suture is started at the head of the pancreas, run along the inferior border of the pancreas toward the middle in a similar fashion, and tied to the first suture.
- The superior aspect of the pancreaticojejunostomy is sutured in a similar fashion (Figure 12-8).

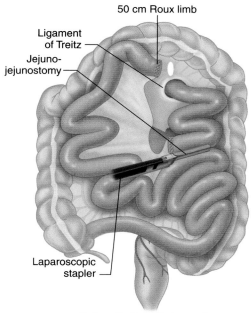

Figure 12-6

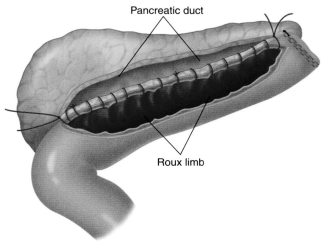

Figure 12-7

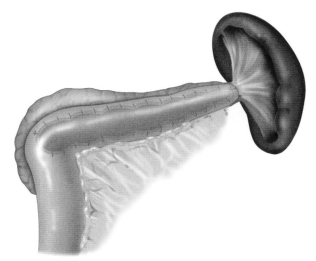

Figure 12-8

Closure

- Suction drains are placed along the superior and inferior borders of the anastomosis and brought out through the port sites.
- The Nathanson retractor is removed.
- The ports are removed under direct vision, and pneumoperitoneum is deflated.
- Skin incisions are closed in the usual fashion.

Step 4. Postoperative Care

- Patients are provided with a patient-controlled analgesia (PCA), and the nasogastric tube is kept in overnight.
- After removal of the nasogastric tube on the first postoperative day, the patients are given sips and then advanced to liquids the next day.
- The expected hospital stay is 4 to 5 days.
- Drains should be kept in until there is low output.

Step 5. Pearls and Pitfalls

- This is an uncommon procedure with few published reports. Most described techniques are similar to what has been described here.[3-5]
- Previous history of recurrent attacks of pancreatitis can make entry into the lesser sac difficult, and care should be taken during this part.
- Conversion to open surgery should be considered when anatomic landmarks and structures are not clear, and palpation is thought to help in this process.
- The pancreatic tissue is usually thick, and thus the likelihood of pancreatic leak is relatively low.

Selected References

Hines O, Reber H: *Chronic pancreatitis.* In Zinner M, Ashley S (editors): *Maingot's Abdominal Operations,* ed 11, Chap. 8. New York, McGraw Hill, 2007.

Cahen DL, Gouma DJ, Nio Y, et al: *Endoscopic versus surgical drainage of the pancreatic duct in chronic pancreatitis.* N Engl J Med 356(7): 676-84, 2007.

Kurian MS, Gagner M: *Laparoscopic side-to-side pancreaticojejunostomy (Partington-Rochelle) for chronic pancreatitis.* J Hepatobiliary Pancreat Surg 6(4):382-86, 1999.

Palanivelu C, Shetty R, Jani K, et al: *Laparoscopic lateral pancreaticojejunostomy: a new remedy for an old ailment.* Surg Endosc 20(3):458-61, 2006.

Tantia O, Jindal MK, Khanna S, et al: *Laparoscopic lateral pancreaticojejunostomy: our experience of 17 cases.* Surg Endosc 18(7):1054-57, 2004.

13

SPLENECTOMY

Lily Chang and Fru Bahiraei

Step 1. Surgical Anatomy

- The spleen is mobilized by dividing the splenic attachments and ligating the vascular hilum without injury to the nearby stomach or pancreatic tail.
- Peritoneal attachments and splenic ligaments can be divided using electrocautery or ultrasonic cutting devices.
- The vascular supply requires adequate ligation for proper hemostasis. This can be achieved using energy devices as well as vessel sealing systems, clips, and laparoscopic staplers.

Step 2. Preoperative Considerations

Patient Preparation

- It is important to consider spleen size when preparing a patient for laparoscopic splenectomy. This will determine the port placement as well as the potential need for a hand-assist port.
- Any evidence of an accessory spleen seen on preoperative imaging should be noted, particularly for hematologic indications for splenectomy.
- Patients with idiopathic thrombocytopenic purpura (ITP) and a preoperative platelet count less than 20,000 should be prepared for intraoperative platelet transfusion. Steroids and intravenous immunoglobulin can be given prior to surgery to temporarily elevate the platelet count.
- While the risk for overwhelming postsplenectomy infections (OPSI) is small, it is advised that vaccinations be given 2 to 3 weeks prior to an elective operation. These should include vaccinations for encapsulated organisms: *Streptococcus Pneumoniae, Haemophilus Influenza B*, and *Neisseria Meningitidis*.
- Hand assistance may be helpful in cases of splenomegaly or when removal of an intact specimen is needed.

Equipment and Instrumentation

- Standard laparoscopic instrumentation is required, including abdominal access devices (e.g., Veress needle or visualization ports), 12-mm and 5-mm ports; 30-degree endoscope; standard laparoscopic instruments including scissors, graspers, and electrocautery; suction-irrigator; and large endoscopic specimen retrieval bag.
- Specialized equipment is also necessary for vessel ligation and hemostasis. A variety of devices can be used, including laparoscopic staplers with vascular loads, clip appliers, ultrasonic coagulation, or bipolar electrocoagulation devices.
- Laparoscopic ultrasound may be helpful in locating accessory spleens or identification of vascular supply.

Anesthetic

- Laparoscopic splenectomy is performed under general anesthesia.
- Typically, sequential compression devices (SCDs) are placed on the lower extremities for deep venous thrombosis (DVT) prophylaxis.
- Preoperative antibiotics should be administered. A first-generation cephalosporin, such as cefazolin, is appropriate.
- A nasogastric tube is used to decompress the stomach during surgery, but it may be removed at the end of the operation.
- A Foley catheter can be placed before surgery and removed at the conclusion if a prolonged operative time is expected.
- Invasive monitoring is typically not needed for elective cases unless the patient has significant underlying cardiopulmonary disease.
- Platelets should be available for transfusion if patient is severely thrombocytopenic (<20,000).

Positioning

- The patient is placed in the right lateral decubitus position.
- Flexion of the operating table improves access. The kidney rest can also be used to increase the space between the costal margin and the anterior superior iliac spine.
- Stabilization of the patient's position can be achieved using a beanbag device or rolls on either side of the patient.
- The reverse Trendelenburg position may aid with exposure of the hilum.
- Both the surgeon and the assistant typically stand on the right side of patient.
- The surgeon needs to be prepared for the possibility of conversion to an open procedure through a left subcostal or midline incision when placing the drapes.

Step 3. Operative Steps

Access and Port Placement

- A Veress needle is inserted through a small left subcostal incision for insufflation, unless there are left upper quadrant adhesions or a prohibitively large spleen.
- Using a 30-degree endoscope greatly facilitates visualization.
- Once the camera and ports are introduced, a visual examination of the abdomen is made to search for access injuries and accessory spleens.

- ◆ The objective is to triangulate the ports (camera and working instruments) around the spleen:
  - ▲ 12-mm port left-superior periumbilical (camera port)
  - ▲ 5-mm or 12-mm port left epigastrium (surgeon's left hand)
  - ▲ 12-mm left anterior axillary line, subcostal (surgeon's right hand)
  - ▲ 5-mm left midaxillary line, subcostal (assistant retraction) (Figure 13-1)

Description of Procedure

Splenic Flexure Mobilization

- ◆ The first step is to mobilize the splenic flexure of the colon medially by incising the splenocolic ligament. To avoid colonic injury, electrocautery is used sparingly (Figure 13-2).
- ◆ Entry into Gerota's fascia posteriorly should be avoided.
- ◆ The gastrosplenic ligament and short gastric vessels are best divided with appropriate energy devices or ultrasonic coagulation.
- ◆ The splenophrenic ligament provides excellent lateral retraction of the spleen and should be left intact until the final steps of the procedure.
- ◆ The spleen is then elevated, exposing the vascular hilum medially.
- ◆ Hilar vessels are ligated and divided using electrocautery, ultrasonic shears, hand ties, or staplers. These devices can also be used in combination depending on the size of the vessels and hilar vascular anatomy (Figure 13-3).
- ◆ Care is taken to avoid injury to the pancreatic tail.
- ◆ When possible, the artery is ligated first, followed by the vein, but this often depends upon hilar anatomy.
- ◆ Once the hilum is divided, the posterior and lateral attachments are divided.

Removal of Spleen

- ◆ The approach for splenic removal will depend on size and pathology. Usually the spleen is placed into an endoscopic bag, and the opening of the bag is brought through the left subcostal port site with extension of the incision or hand port incision, if present.
- ◆ The spleen is morcellated within the bag using ringed forceps and removed piecemeal.
- ◆ Care must be taken not to rupture the bag or spill splenic tissue into the peritoneal cavity.
- ◆ A larger spleen that needs to be examined intact may require the surgeon to extend the incision, or connect two incisions, for extraction.

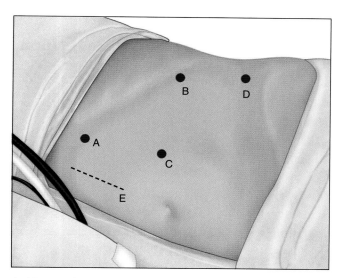

A, 12 mm epigastric port for surgeon's left hand
B, 12 mm left subcostal port for surgeon's right hand
C, 12 mm camera port periumbilical
D, 5 mm port for assistant
E, upper midline hand asistant port (if needed)
   would replace (A)

Figure 13-1

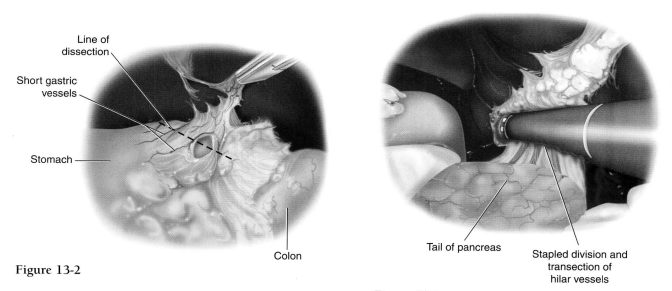

Figure 13-2

Figure 13-3

Closure

- No drains are needed unless there is suspicion for pancreatic injury.
- A fascial closure device may be used to reapproximate the fascia of the larger incisions.
- Final laparoscopic inspection is performed to ensure no inadvertent injuries have occurred and hemostasis is present.

Step 4. Postoperative Care

- Patients are typically admitted to the hospital for 1 to 2 days postoperatively for recovery.
- Nasogastric decompression is not necessary in most patients.
- Postoperative hematocrit or platelet count may be checked.
- A liquid diet is initiated on postoperative day 1 and advanced as tolerated.
- Pain management generally includes patient-controlled analgesia (PCA) with or without nonsteroidal anti-inflammatory agents.

Step 5. Pearls and Pitfalls

- Clips should be avoided near the hilar vessels because they can become caught within a stapling device and will result in an inadequate deployment of staples.
- Platelet transfusion should occur after the artery is ligated to provide maximum benefit and avoid sequestration.
- The inspection for any accessory spleens should occur at the beginning of the procedure prior to disruption of the field.
- The specimen retrieval bag should be monitored with the laparoscope during morcellation to avoid rupture.

Selected References

George JN, Woolf SH, Raskob GE, et al: Idiopathic thrombocytopenic purpura: a practice guideline developed by explicit methods for the American Society of Hematology.*Blood* 88(1):3-40, 1996.
Keidar A, Feldman M, Szold A: Analysis of outcome of laparoscopic splenectomy for idiopathic thrombocytopenic purpura by platelet count. *Am J Hematol* 80(2):95-100, 2005.
Schilling RF: Estimating the risk for sepsis after splenectomy in hereditary spherocytosis. *Ann Intern Med* 122(3):187-88, 1995.

14

ADRENALECTOMY

L. Michael Brunt and Corey Ming-Lum

Step 1. Surgical Anatomy

A thorough knowledge of normal adrenal anatomy and the relationship of the adrenals to surrounding structures is essential for surgeons who undertake adrenalectomy.

- The adrenal glands are located at the superior-medial aspect of each kidney and are composed of a cortex and medulla with distinct endocrine functions. The steroid hormones (cortisol, aldosterone, and the adrenal androgens) are synthesized and secreted in the adrenal cortex, and the adrenal medulla synthesizes the catecholamines, norepinephrine and epinephrine. Catecholamines may also be synthesized in extra-adrenal chromaffin tissue in the paraganglia.
- Each adrenal gland is embedded in Gerota's fascia and is surrounded by retroperitoneal fat. The adrenal gland has a golden yellow appearance because of the high lipid content of the cortex.
- The *right* adrenal gland is pyramidal in shape and lies superior to the right kidney, whereas the *left* adrenal is more flattened and is in intimate contact with the medial aspect of the superior pole of the left kidney.
- Bordering structures for the *right* adrenal are the inferior vena cava medially, the liver anteriorly, and the kidney inferiorly. A portion of the anteromedial border of the gland usually extends posterior to the vena cava. The right triangular ligament of the liver crosses the anterior surface of the adrenal gland superiorly, which means that the upper portion of the gland has no peritoneum covering its surface. Structures that border the posterior aspect of the *right* adrenal are the diaphragm superiorly and the anteromedial portion of the superior pole of the right kidney inferiorly.
- Structures neighboring the *left* adrenal gland are the spleen and fundus of the stomach superiorly, the splenic flexure of the colon, the tail of pancreas, and splenic vessels inferiorly, and the left crus of the diaphragm posteromedially and the medial aspect of the left kidney posterolaterally. The renal vessels lie just below the inferior border of the adrenal, and in the setting of a large tumor, they may overlie the renal artery and vein.
- The adrenal blood supply is derived from numerous branches of the inferior phrenic, aortic, and renal arteries. A single central vein drains each adrenal.
  - ▲ The *right* adrenal vein is short (0.5 to 1 cm in length) and runs from the medial aspect of the gland directly into the posterolateral aspect of the inferior vena cava. A second *right* adrenal vein may occasionally enter either the vena cava or right hepatic vein more superiorly.

▲ The *left* adrenal vein is longer than on the right (2 to 3 cm in length) and is found at the inferior-medial aspect of the gland, where it runs obliquely to empty into the left renal vein. The inferior phrenic vein typically joins the left adrenal vein proximal to its entry into the renal vein (Figure 14-1).

Step 2. Preoperative Considerations

◆ Most indications for adrenalectomy today are appropriate for a laparoscopic approach. The only absolute contraindication for laparoscopic adrenalectomy is an adrenal malignancy with evidence of local invasion or involved regional lymph nodes. However, surgeons should be cautious in approaching large tumors laparoscopically for a number of reasons: (1) large tumors are more difficult to remove, (2) the tumor is more likely to be malignant (especially adrenal cortical lesions >6 cm in size), and (3) the surgeon should be highly experienced in laparoscopic adrenalectomy.
◆ All patients undergoing adrenalectomy should have completed a biochemical evaluation to assess for a functioning tumor. The minimal workup should consist of the following:
  ▲ Plasma fractionated metanephrines or 24-hour urine catecholamines and metanephrines to exclude a pheochromocytoma
  ▲ Overnight dexamethasone test (1 mg dexamethasone at 11 PM followed by 8 AM plasma cortisol) to rule out hypercortisolism; plasma cortisol should suppress to <3 µg/dL in normal subjects
  ▲ Plasma aldosterone and renin levels in patients who are hypertensive or hypokalemic to exclude an aldosteronoma

Preoperative preparation for adrenalectomy should entail the following:
◆ Control of hypertension and correction of any electrolyte abnormalities.
◆ Pharmacologic preparation of patients with pheochromocytomas with alpha-adrenergic blockade for 7 to 10 days preoperatively to mitigate against hypertensive exacerbations intraoperatively. Most commonly, phenoxybenzamine is used starting at 10 mg twice daily, with the dose increasing until hypertension and tachycardia are controlled and the patient is mildly orthostatic.

Equipment and Instrumentation

◆ Laparoscopic adrenalectomy is carried out with standard laparoscopic dissecting instruments, atraumatic graspers, and a hook electrocautery.
◆ Additional equipment that facilitates the procedure may include the following:
  ▲ Ultrasonic or bipolar coagulating device
  ▲ Right angle dissector
  ▲ Specimen retrieval bag
  ▲ Laparoscopic ultrasound (optional)—may be useful for larger tumors or in obese patients if there is difficulty in locating the adrenal

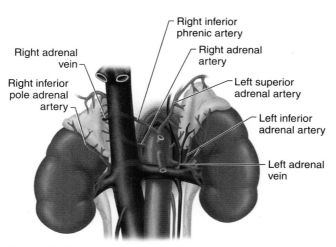

Figure 14-1

Anesthesia

- Our usual protocol includes a single dose of first-generation cephalosporin prior to skin incision.
- A nasogastric tube is usually unnecessary.
- A Foley catheter is only used in patients in whom a longer procedure is expected (i.e., for pheos and large tumors over 5 cm).
- Stress-dose steroids are administered for patients with Cushing syndrome or those undergoing bilateral adrenalectomy. Steroids are tapered to maintenance doses early postoperatively and are continued until recovery of the pituitary-adrenal axis.

Room Setup and Patient Positioning

- The transabdominal lateral flank approach is the most commonly utilized laparoscopic approach. Some centers favor a direct retroperitoneal endoscopic approach with the patient in a prone position.
- Sequential steps in the transabdominal lateral approach are as follows:
  - ▲ The patient is in a lateral decubitus position with the affected side up (Figure 14-2).
  - ▲ A beanbag mattress that is well padded is used to secure the patient to the operating table. A roll is placed under the chest to protect the axilla.
  - ▲ The legs are wrapped with a foam egg crate roll and secured around the table with tape.

Step 3. Operative Steps

Access and Port Placement

- Initial access is obtained by closed Veress needle insertion and insufflation in the subcostal region just medial to the anterior axillary line. An optical 5-mm trocar is used for initial access, and the other ports are placed under direct laparoscopic visualization. Alternatively, an open insertion technique can be used (Figure 14-3).
- The ports should be at least 5 cm apart to allow external freedom of movement. One of the ports is 10 to 12 mm in size (usually the midaxillary port) for insertion of the clip applier and specimen extraction, and the others are 5 mm in diameter.

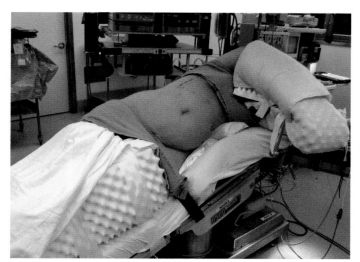

Figure 14-2

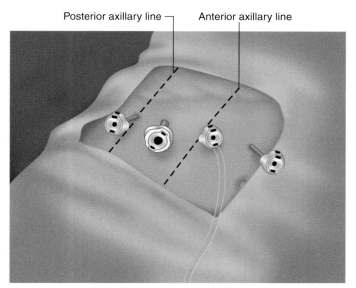

Posterior axillary line   Anterior axillary line

Figure 14-3

Right Adrenalectomy

Mobilization of Liver

The first step in right adrenalectomy is mobilization of the right lobe of the liver by division of the right triangular ligament. This maneuver can be done with either the hook cautery or an ultrasonic or bipolar energy device. The ligament should be divided all the way to the diaphragm to allow medial rotation of the liver off the adrenal and vena cava. A 5-mm retractor is used to retract the liver medially once the ligament has been divided.

Dissection of Medial Border of the Adrenal

The peritoneum between the liver and the right adrenal is incised and the plane is developed between the adrenal and the inferior vena cava. The adrenal is gently retracted medially and small arterial branches to the middle and upper adrenal are hooked and cauterized. The adrenal vein should come into view early in the dissection (Figure 14-4).

Division of Right Adrenal Vein

The adrenal vein is isolated, clipped, and divided. A right-angle dissector is used to get around the vein. The vein is short and care must be taken to not exert much traction on it as it may tear at its junction with the vena cava (Figure 14-5).

Inferior Adrenal Dissection

The medial border of the adrenal is freed up down to the underlying back muscle, and the dissection is extended inferiorly. The inferior portion of the adrenal sits on top of the kidney and extends toward the renal vessels. The dissection is carried inferiorly and then laterally out over the superior pole of the kidney, dividing the perinephric fat. Either a hook cautery or an ultrasonic device may be used for this portion of the dissection, and clips are applied to any larger vessels. The dissection should stay close to the inferior adrenal pole because of the proximity of the renal hilum and superior pole arterial branches (Figure 14-6).

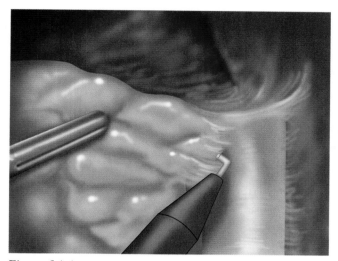

Figure 14-4

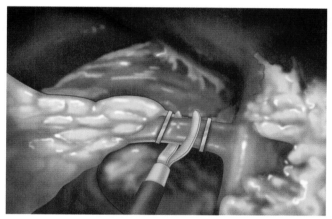

Figure 14-5

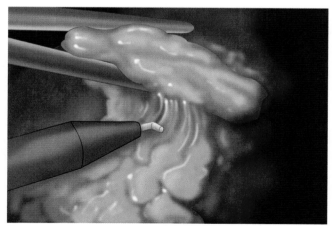

Figure 14-6

Lateral and Posterior Dissection

The adrenal is elevated off the top of the kidney, and the remaining lateral and posterior attachments are divided.

Specimen Removal

The retroperitoneum is irrigated and inspected for hemostasis. The adrenal is then placed in an impermeable entrapment bag for removal. Small tumors may be removed intact within the bag by enlarging the incision and fascial opening somewhat. For larger tumors in which pathologic margins are not important (e.g., pheochromocytomas), we prefer to morcellate the specimen within the bag and remove it piecemeal so as to avoid making a large incision.

Wound Closure

The fascia at the extraction site is closed under direct vision with a 0-gauge polygolic absorbable suture. The skin at the extraction site is closed with 4-0 monofilament absorbable suture, and the 5 mm incision sites are steri-stripped.

Left Adrenalectomy

Take Down of Splenic Flexure of Colon

The first step in left adrenalectomy is mobilization of the splenic flexure of the colon. This should be released from the lateral abdominal reflection all the way to the inferior pole of the spleen (Figure 14-7).

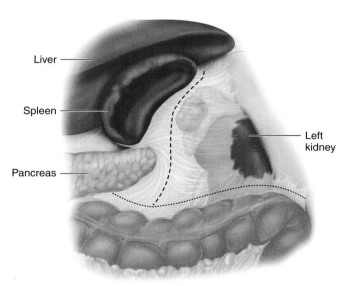

Liver

Spleen

Pancreas

Left
kidney

Figure 14-7

Division of Splenorenal Ligament and Mobilization of Tail of Pancreas

The splenorenal ligament is divided to the diaphragm with an ultrasonic coagulator or bipolar coagulating/cutting device to allow full medial rotation. The tail of the pancreas should come into view at this point, and the plane between the pancreas and the kidney is then developed staying just lateral to the pancreas. The splenic artery and vein are often visible at this point in the dissection. Entering this plane is key to exposure of the adrenal, which should come into view as the dissection proceeds cephalad.

Dissection of Medial and Lateral Borders of Adrenal

Once the adrenal is visualized, the lateral and medial borders are defined and freed up with ultrasonic or cautery dissection. Small arterial branches entering the medial and lateral adrenal are divided with ultrasonic or bipolar energy. The dissection then proceeds to delineate the inferior border of the adrenal. The renal vein lies just below the inferior adrenal, and with large inferior pole tumors, the adrenal may actually overlie the renal vein.

Isolation and Division of Left Adrenal Vein

The adrenal vein exits the adrenal obliquely at the inferior-medial border of the gland. The surrounding small vessels and connective tissue are dissected with the hook cautery and the vein is isolated with a right angle dissector. It is clipped and then divided (Figure 14-8).

Posterior and Superior Dissection

Once the adrenal vein has been divided, the inferior adrenal is gently elevated, and it is taken off the posterior diaphragm and the medial left kidney with an ultrasonic coagulator.

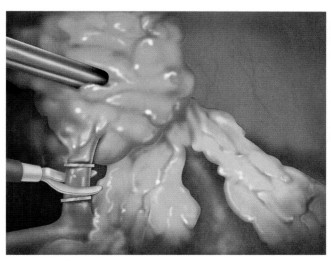

Figure 14-8

Specimen Removal and Wound Closure

The retroperitoneum is irrigated, inspected for hemostasis, and the specimen is removed as described for right adrenalectomy. The wounds are closed in a similar manner as well.

Step 4. Postoperative Care

- Day of surgery: Patients are admitted to a regular nursing unit and are started on a liquid diet once they are awake and alert. Exceptions are patients with vasoactive pheochromocytomas who may require a period of postoperative pressor support with arterial line monitoring, in which case they should be monitored in an intensive care unit setting.
- Postoperative day 1: Serum electrolytes and creatinine are obtained and the diet is advanced. Patients may be discharged once blood pressure is stable and they are tolerating a regular diet. Some patients may require longer in-hospital monitoring for blood pressure management or adjustments in hormone replacement.
- Patients with Cushing syndrome should receive perioperative stress steroids tapered rapidly to maintenance levels. For bilateral adrenalectomy, patients should receive both prednisone and mineralocorticoid replacement with fludrocortisone (0.1 mg/dL).
- Patients with aldosteronomas should have the spironolactone stopped, and other antihypertensive medications should be continued and subsequently adjusted or discontinued as clinically indicated.

Step 5. Pearls and Pitfalls

- Surgeons who undertake adrenalectomy should be well versed in the biochemical evaluation of adrenal tumors and in options for adrenal imaging.
- A thorough knowledge of adrenal anatomy and relationships of surrounding structures is essential to successful adrenalectomy.
- A gentle, meticulous dissection technique should be used to minimize operative bleeding, to maintain clear dissection planes, and to avoid fracturing the adrenal capsule or tumor.
- Difficult cases (pheochromocytoma, obese patients, those with large tumors) should be avoided early in one's experience with adrenalectomy.
- Large, malignant adrenal cortical cancers should be removed in an open fashion.

Selected References

Brunt LM: *Minimal access adrenal surgery. Surg Endosc* 20(3):351-61, 2006.

Brunt LM, Moley JF: *Adrenal incidentaloma.* In Cameron JL (editor): *Current Surgical Therapy,* ed 9, St. Louis, Mosby, 2008, pp. 597-602.

Duh Q-Y, Inabnet WB, Brunt LM: *SAGES Grand Rounds Master Series Episode VII: Adrenal Tumors.* SAGES—Cine-Med, Woodbury, CT, 2008.

Tessier D, Brunt LM: *Laparoscopic adrenalectomy.* In Soper NJ, Swanstrom LL, Eubanks, WS (editors): *Mastery of Endoscopic and Laparoscopic Surgery,* 3rd ed. Philadelphia, Lippincott, Williams & Wilkins, 2009, pp. 410-420.

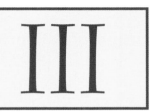

Abdominal Wall Surgery

15

TOTAL EXTRAPERITONEAL (TEP) HERNIA REPAIR

Patricia Sylla and David W. Rattner

Step 1. Surgical Anatomy

- A thorough knowledge of the extraperitoneal inguinal anatomy is required to avoid complications. The most important first step for successful completion of total extraperitoneal (TEP) hernia repair is correct entry into the preperitoneal space. Upon dissection of the preperitoneal space, proper orientation is confirmed by visualizing the rectus abdominis muscles superiorly, the preperitoneal fat and peritoneum inferiorly, the pubic symphysis and Cooper's ligament in the midline, and the inferior epigastric vessels laterally (Figure 15-1).

Step 2. Preoperative Considerations

Patient Selection

- Relative to standard open inguinal herniorrhaphy, the laparoscopic approach provides superb laparoscopic visualization of the inguinal anatomy with magnified views, with the added benefit of being able to evaluate and repair the contralateral side without the need for additional incisions. Relative to open hernia repair, the laparoscopic approach is associated with improved cosmesis, reduced postoperative pain, faster recovery and return to work, and similar complication and recurrence rates. In the setting of a recurrent inguinal hernia following previous open repair, a laparoscopic repair is the preferred approach. Not only does it avoid dissection through old scar, but it is associated with reduced postoperative and recovery time and similar or improved recurrence rates compared with reoperative open herniorrhaphy.

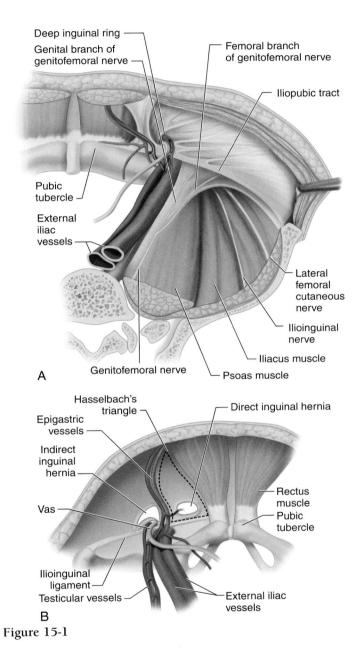

A

B

Figure 15-1

- Laparoscopic repair can be performed either transabdominally (TAPP) or totally extraperitoneally (TEP); the choice largely depends on the surgeon's experience and preference.
- Relative to TAPP, TEP, which is performed without violating the peritoneal space, may reduce the incidence of postoperative adhesions.
- Absolute contraindications to laparoscopic inguinal hernia repair include any medical condition that precludes general anesthesia, such as severe cardiac or pulmonary disease. Other contraindications include incarcerated and potentially strangulated hernia. Relative contraindications include previous prostatic surgery, which will distort anatomic planes. In addition, TEP repair may complicate future prostatic surgery, which should be a consideration for older male patients.

Preoperative Preparation and Anesthetic Considerations

- Patients are instructed to void just prior to the procedure to minimize the use of urinary catheters. The combination of excessive intraoperative fluids and bladder catherization can be associated with an increased incidence of urinary retention. DVT prophylaxis is not required unless the patient is at risk for thromboembolism.
- Following general endotracheal anesthesia and muscle paralysis, the abdomen is shaved, prepped with antiseptic solution, and draped using a Steri-Drape. Prophylactic antibiotics are administered intravenously. First-generation cephalosporin or vancomycin in penicillin-allergic patients is typically given preoperatively. Patients are placed supine on the table with arms either positioned to the sides or tucked.

Surgical Equipment

◆ Laparoscopic instrumentation includes a 30-degree, 10-mm laparoscopic camera; two 5-mm trocars; two blunt graspers; a 5-mm laparoscopic tacker; and one or two 6-by-6-inch pieces of polypropylene mesh.
◆ We prefer using a 10-mm dilating trocar for dissection, as opposed to blunt dissection, and a 10-mm structural trocar with pump for balloon inflation.
◆ Laparoscopic suction and diathermy should be available.

Operating Room Setup

◆ The operating surgeon stands on the opposite side of the hernia with the assistant holding the camera across the table. The laparoscopic monitors and instrument tray should be positioned at the feet of the operating table.

Step 3. Operative Steps

Entry and Dissection of the Preperitoneal Space

◆ A 2- to 3-cm transverse incision is made with a skin knife just lateral and below the umbilicus on the side opposite the symptomatic hernia. This incision avoids the midline where the anterior and posterior rectus sheaths merge. This incision is carried down through the subcutaneous tissues down to the anterior rectus sheath, which is incised with a 15-mm blade, just enough to expose the underlying rectus muscle. This incision is extended on either side with Metzenbaum scissors. The curved Mayo scissors are used to retract the rectus muscle laterally to expose the underlying posterior sheath (Figure 15-2).

- The surgeon carefully inserts the 10-mm dilating trocar in the space underneath the rectus muscle on top of the posterior rectus sheath and advances it inferiorly toward the pubic symphysis, making sure to stay away from the midline and maintaining downward traction on the trocar to avoid accidental posterior entry into the peritoneal cavity or bladder injury. The trocar is advanced inferiorly until it reaches the pubic bone in the midline (Figure 15-3).
- The laparoscope is introduced through the trocar, and the balloon is inflated using 40 squeezes of the pump, which instills approximately 1 liter of air. Balloon insufflation of the preperitoneal space is performed under laparoscopic visualization to ensure that the proper plane has been entered (Figure 15-4).
- An alternative for preperitoneal dissection is blunt rather than balloon dissection. The preperitoneal space can be dissected using the laparoscope itself by sweeping it side to side and then placing a standard 10-mm Hassan trocar through the subumbilical incision.
- If proper entry into the preperitoneal space has been achieved, several anatomic landmarks can usually be visualized, including the pubic symphysis in the midline, the rectus muscles anteriorly, and the inferior epigastric vessels laterally (Figure 15-5).

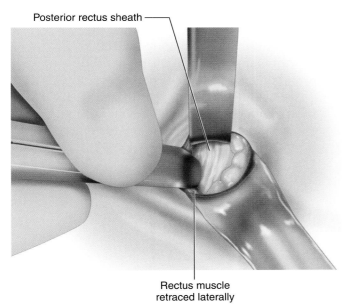

Posterior rectus sheath

Rectus muscle
retraced laterally

Figure 15-2

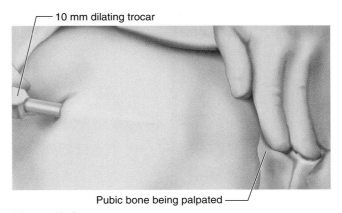

10 mm dilating trocar

Pubic bone being palpated

Figure 15-3

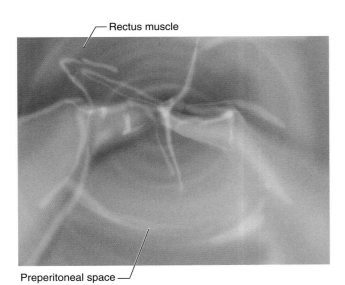

Rectus muscle

Preperitoneal space

Figure 15-4

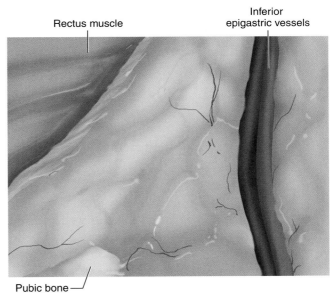

Rectus muscle

Inferior
epigastric vessels

Pubic bone

Figure 15-5

- Following balloon dissection of the preperitoneal space, the balloon is deflated, and the dilating trocar is removed and replaced with the shorter 10-mm structural trocar. The balloon at the tip of the structural trocar is inflated with four squeezes of the pump, and the trocar is locked into position and connected to carbon dioxide, which is insufflated to a pressure of 9 mmHg (Figure 15-6).
- The laparoscope is introduced through the 10-mm structural trocar, and two 5-mm trocars are inserted under laparoscopic visualization, one above the pubic symphysis and the other halfway between the subumbilical and suprapubic ports (Figure 15-7).

Identification of Anatomic Landmarks

- The next step is identification and clearance of the pubic symphysis and Cooper's ligament, which usually requires light blunt dissection of the areolar tissue still obscuring them.
- Using the blunt graspers and following the principles of traction and countertraction, the preperitoneal tissues are bluntly mobilized off the anterior abdominal wall to open up the preperitoneal space further. If not already visualized during balloon dissection, the inferior epigastric vessels should be identified early to avoid inadvertent injury during dissection and to help identify direct and indirect defects.
- Care must be taken to avoid aggressive dissection in the retropubic space and lateral and inferior to Cooper's ligament where the femoral space and iliac vessels are located.

Clearance of the Lateral Space

- The next step consists in the clearance of the lateral space both to complete dissection of the preperitoneal space as well as to prepare for lateral mesh placement. This is performed by bluntly pulling the peritoneum reflection inferiorly, which can usually be visualized as a white edge of peritoneum, and away from the anterior abdominal wall all the way toward the anterior superior iliac spine.

Tip of inflated balloon

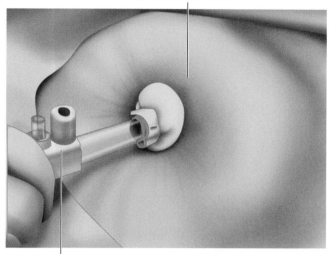

10 mm structural trocar

Figure 15-6

5 mm laparoscopic trocar   Rectus muscle

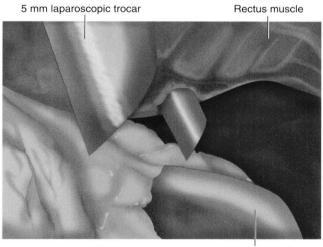

Pubic symphysis

Figure 15-7

Identification of a Direct Defect

♦ During balloon or blunt dissection of the preperitoneal space, if present, a direct hernia is usually reduced. A direct defect can be found just medial to the superficial epigastric vessels, which may be associated with a "pseudosac." This pseudosac, which looks like peritoneum, represents posterior protrusion of the transversalis fascia and needs to be bluntly dissected off preperitoneal fat until it retracts back through the direct defect (Figures 15-8 and 15-9).

Identification of an Indirect Defect

♦ The spermatic cord and round ligament are found just lateral to the inferior epigastric vessels and need to be carefully dissected to identify an indirect sac or lipoma of the cord.
♦ When identified, the sac or lipoma needs to be reduced out of the ring if a scrotal component of the hernia exists. The sac is dissected off the cord structures or round ligament and pulled back, well below the spermatic cord and round ligament (Figure 15-10).
♦ In a man, the dissection is considered complete when the sac is free where the vas and cord structures separate.
♦ Care must be taken to avoid making a hole in the sac during this dissection, which could result in pneumoperitoneum and significant loss of working space. In this event, the defect in the peritoneum can be closed using an Endoloop. Alternatively, a Veress needle can be inserted into the abdominal cavity to evacuate the pneumoperitoneum.

Placement of the Mesh

♦ A 6-by-6-inch piece of polypropylene mesh is trimmed to 4 by 6 inches. The medial lower corner is cut obliquely to mark the level where the mesh should lie medially over Cooper's ligament. Just distal to the oblique cut, a notch is made through the mesh to accommodate the spermatic cord around the mesh.
♦ The mesh is then rolled tightly from medial to lateral, inserted through the structural trocar, and pushed in position using the laparoscope. It is then carefully unrolled and positioned to cover the inguinal floor.
♦ Care should be taken to ensure that the peritoneum and sac (when present) remain below the mesh. The mesh should be positioned such that it covers the direct, indirect, and femoral spaces with good overlap (Figure 15-11).
♦ Once properly positioned, tacks are placed to secure the mesh into position. Typically, a total of three to five tacks are placed: one at the pubic tubercle, another one just distal along Cooper's ligament, and one to three tacks just superior to the pubic tubercle onto the anterior abdominal wall. The lateral component of the mesh is held in place easily by the peritoneum as the carbon dioxide is released.
♦ To avoid injury to the ilioinguinal or genitofemoral nerves, care is taken to avoid placing tacks lateral to the epigastric vessels.

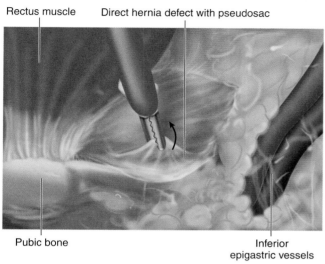

Rectus muscle   Direct hernia defect with pseudosac

Pubic bone   Inferior
                              epigastric vessels

Figure 15-8

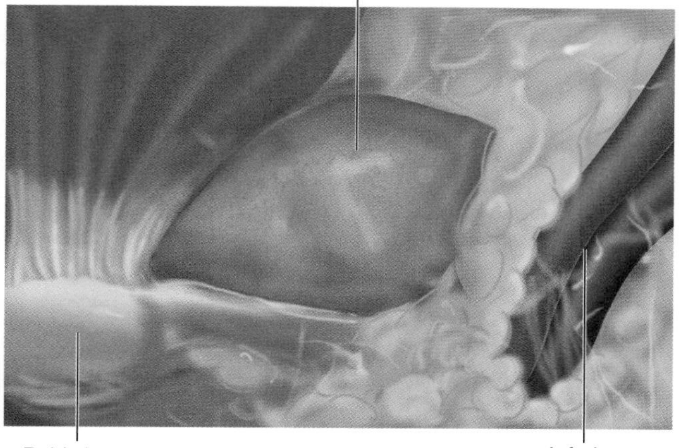

Direct hernia defect after
the pseudosac has been reduced

Pubic bone   Inferior
                              epigastric vessels

Figure 15-9

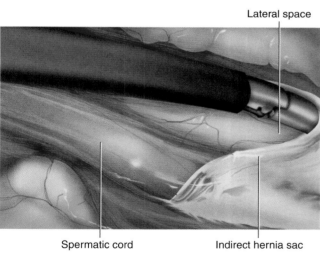

                                          Lateral space

Spermatic cord   Indirect hernia sac

Figure 15-10

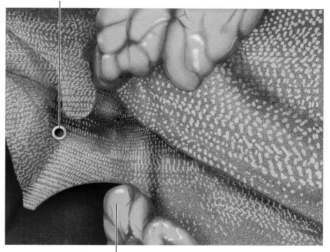

Inferomedial tack placed
along Cooper's ligament

Spermatic cord going
through notch in mesh

Figure 15-11

Wound Closure

- The balloon on the structural trocar is deflated and all ports are removed. The anterior fascia of subumbilical port is closed using a O-Vicryl figure-of-eight suture.
- All skin incisions are infiltrated with local anesthetic and closed using 4-0 Vicryl sutures.
- Steri-Strips and dry dressing are applied to all wounds.

Step 4. Postoperative Management and Instructions

- Patients are discharged home on the day of surgery after voiding. There are no restrictions in physical activities, and patients should expect to be able to return to their baseline activities in 2 to 3 weeks.

Step 5. Pearls and Pitfalls

- Accidental entry into the peritoneal cavity is not by itself an indication to convert the procedure to open repair. The surgeon has several alternatives. One alternative is to re-attempt entry into the proper space through that same incision. Another is to make a second incision on the opposite side of the umbilicus and go through the same steps to enter the preperitoneal plane. If both approaches fail, conversion to TAPP or open repair is indicated.
- One important technical point to avoid nerve injury is the avoidance of monopolar cautery and the use of bipolar cautery only medial to the epigastric vessels if and when used. Similarly, tacks should only be placed medial to the epigastric vessels.

Selected References

Arregui ME, Davis CJ, Yucel O, et al: Laparoscopic mesh repair of inguinal hernia using a preperitoneal approach: a preliminary report. *Surg Laparosc Endosc* 2(1):53-58, 1993.

Bringman S, Haglind E, Heikkinen T, et al: Is a balloon dissection beneficial in totally extraperitoneal hernioplasty (TEP)? *Surg Laparosc Endosc* 15(5):322-6, 2001.

Johansson B, Hallerback B, Glise H, et al: Laparoscopic mesh versus open preperitoneal mesh versus conventional technique for inguinal hernia repair: a randomized multicenter trial (SCUR Hernia Repair Study). *Ann Surg* 230(2):225-31, 1999.

Kieturakis MJ, Nguyen DT, Vargas H, et al: Balloon dissection facilitated laparoscopic extraperitoneal hernioplasty. *Am J Surg* 168(6): 603-07, 1994.

McKernan JB, Laws HL: Laparoscopic mesh repair of inguinal hernia using a preperitoneal prosthetic approach. *Surg Endosc* 7(1):26-28, 1993.

Takata MC, Duh QY: Laparoscopic inguinal hernia repair. *Surg Clin N Am* 88(1):157-78, 2008.

Wake BL, McCormack K, Fraser C, et al: Transabdominal preperitoneal (TAPP) vs totally extraperitoneal (TEP) laparoscopic techniques for inguinal hernia repair. *Cochrane Database Syst Rev* 1:CD004703, 2005.

CHAPTER 16

VENTRAL INCISIONAL HERNIA

Robert Lim and Daniel B. Jones

Step 1. Surgical Anatomy

- ◆ Ventral hernia repair is a common operation in the United States. With the realization that mesh is more durable than primary closure alone, fascial defects greater than 3 cm are often repaired with mesh reinforcement. More and more, the laparoscopic approach has gained popularity.
- ◆ The laparoscopic approach may lessen the morbidity by avoiding a laparotomy and lowering the incidence of hernia recurrence by providing wide mesh coverage of the defect. Additionally, direct laparoscopic visualization of the abdominal cavity can help the surgeon to identify "Swiss cheese" multiple fascial defects.

Step 2. Preoperative Considerations

Patient Preparation

- ◆ Because the risk of recurrence is relatively high for these procedures, not all hernias need to be repaired when discovered. Elective repair should be considered for patients who have pain or in whom the hernia has enlarged over time.
- ◆ Patients who have severe pain may need urgent or even emergent surgery to prevent strangulation of bowel. Sharp pain or peritoneal signs suggest the possibility of bowel strangulation or necrosis.
- ◆ Laparoscopic ventral hernia repair requires the use of general anesthesia. Patients need to undergo appropriate preoperative evaluation to determine their ability to tolerate the procedure.
- ◆ A computed tomography (CT) scan may be useful to confirm the diagnosis of hernia or to delineate the size of the hernia when physical exam is difficult, such as in obese patients.

Equipment and Instrumentation

- Standard laparoscopic instrumentation is required, including scissors and atraumatic graspers.
- For access, we prefer using a Veress needle and an optical trocar with a 0-degree endoscope.
- Once the procedure is underway, it is helpful to use a 5-mm, 30-degree endoscope to allow viewing through any of the 5-mm ports. At least one larger port will be required to introduce the mesh into the abdominal cavity.
- Equipment for hemostasis is necessary even though it is used sparingly. It can be helpful to have electrocautery and clip appliers, and in some cases, ultrasonic coagulation can be used for vessel ligation and hemostasis.

Anesthesia

- Sequential compression devices should be placed and subcutaneous heparin should be given for thromboembolic prophylaxis preoperatively.
- Intravenous antibiotics, usually a first-generation cephalosporin, should be administered prophylactically to cover skin flora. Broader coverage for gram-negative organisms may be added in case of an enterotomy.
- Although formal bowel prep is usually not necessary, a bowel prep may be elected at the surgeon's discretion when a difficult lysis of adhesions is anticipated.
- After induction of anesthesia, the stomach and bladder are decompressed with an orogastric and urinary catheter, respectively.
- The abdomen is scrubbed and painted with Betadine. The patient's abdomen may then be covered with Ioban barrier to limit the mesh contact with skin.

Room Setup and Patient Positioning

- The patient is placed in the supine position with arms tucked to facilitate a greater range of movement for the surgeon and assistant around the operative table.
- The surgeon usually stands on the patient's right side with an assistant on the opposite side.
  - ▲ There should be two monitors, one on each side of the table, and they can be positioned at the foot or head of the bed depending on the surgeon's preference.
  - ▲ It is not unusual for the primary surgeon to switch sides of the table in order to better visualize the entire surgical field.

Step 3. Operative Steps

Access and Port Placement

We routinely mark the costal margin, xyphoid process, anterior superior iliac spines, pubic symphysis, previous scars, and hernia prior to insufflation to aid with port placement.

- Pneumoperitoneum can be achieved with either an open or closed technique, but the initial incision should be at least 10 cm away from the closest margin of the defect.

- For a midline abdominal incisional hernia, we will often start with a Veress needle in the left subcostal location. After drop test and insufflation with carbon dioxide to create a pneumoperitoneum, we use a 12-mm optical trocar Visiport (Covidien, Mansfield, Massachusetts) for initial access. This is placed far from the midline incision and the hernia (Figure 16-1).
- After assuring there is no iatrogenic injury with a straight scope, we will switch to an angled scope (30 or 45 degrees) to achieve better visualization. Two subsequent 5-mm ports should be placed under direct visualization in the right and left flanks. While a 5-mm scope can allow viewing from all ports, at least one larger port will be required to introduce the mesh into the abdominal cavity.
- Ports positioned too close to the hernia may affect visualization and access to the hernia.

Reduce Hernia Contents

- Sometimes the hernia will reduce completely with only gentle external pressure on the anterior abdominal wall. More commonly, external pressure aids the dissection. For difficult cases, additional 5-mm ports may be required to achieve adequate countertraction during dissection.
- We limit use of electrocautery and the Harmonic scalpel in an effort to reduce the chance of inadvertent intestinal burn injury. We will reduce enough of the abdominal wall adhesions to allow the wide mesh overlap of the hernia defect.
- In general, we do not excise or invert the hernia sac at operation, but we do discuss with patients preoperatively the likelihood of a postoperative seroma.

Choosing the Size of the Mesh

Once the hernia or hernias are identified, the fascial defect is again marked. We use a spinal needle to identify areas in four quadrants that are 3 to 5 cm outside the hernia defect(s). These points are marked on the patient's abdomen. The surgeon must be careful to introduce this needle perpendicularly for accurate sizing.

- If the hernia size has been overestimated, the mesh may not lay flat and may lead to adhesions or recurrence.
- If too small a mesh is chosen, recurrence may also occur, especially if mesh contracts over time.

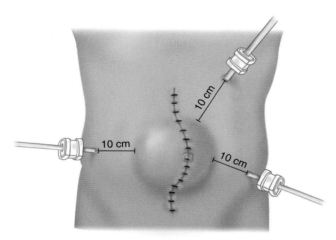

Figure 16-1

Placing the Mesh

Once the size of defect is carefully estimated, we generally choose a mesh that allows a 4-cm mesh overlap of the fascial defect (Figure 16-2).

- We prefer the dual-sided mesh, which promotes healing against the abdominal wall but retards adhesions to its inner surface toward the bowel.
- The mesh is prepared with sutures placed at each corner with 0-Prolene suture. Larger meshes will require additional sutures, and we will use a white Gore suture to help distinguish its tails from the blue Prolene corner sutures.
- The lateral edges of the mesh are then rolled inward like a scrolled letter. The mesh is then inserted through the 12-mm port site. Alternatively, the mesh can also be delivered by using a grasper from a separate port site to pull it into the abdomen (Figure 16-3).
- For larger meshes, the 12-mm port can be removed, and the rolled mesh is directly passed through the abdominal wall port site.

Fixing the Mesh to the Wall

- The mesh is unrolled ensuring that the porous side is facing the abdominal wall and the smooth side of mesh faces the bowel beneath (Figure 16-4).
- A 2-mm incision is made on the skin at one of the corner points marked on the patient's abdomen.
  - ▲ The tails of the corresponding suture are then pulled up through the abdominal wall using a fascial closure device. The sutures are not tied until is it certain that the defect is well covered and that the mesh will lay flat (Figure 16-5).
  - ▲ Tension is kept on the mesh by placing a crile or mosquito clamp on the suture tails. The remaining three sutures are grasped in a similar manner.
  - ▲ Once the mesh can be pulled taut and adequate coverage is ensured, the sutures are tied in the subcutaneous tissue to provide four-point transabdominal fixation (Figure 16-6).

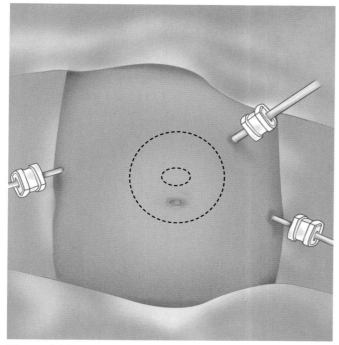

Figure 16-2

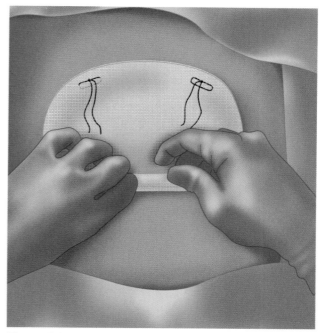

Figure 16-3

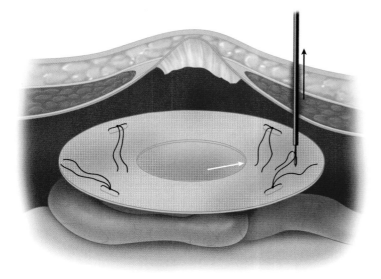

Figure 16-4

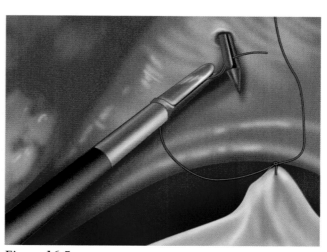

Figure 16-5

- After suture fixation is achieved, the mesh is stapled to the abdominal wall using a 5-mm spiral tacking device. The insufflation pressure is decreased to 12 mmHg and external manual counter pressure is applied to the abdominal wall so the stapler fires straight into the abdominal wall.
  - ▲ The tacks are placed at 1- to 2-cm intervals at the edge of the mesh to prevent small bowel from slipping between the mesh and the abdominal wall. Until recently, spiral tacks have been made of titanium. New tacks are made of synthetic materials and will absorb over time. The absorbable tacks are currently reserved for mesh less than 1 mm in thickness (Figure 16-7).
  - ▲ If more transabdominal fixation is needed, additional sutures can be deployed using a fascial closure device that is passed directly through the abdominal wall and the underlying mesh. These are done through separate small skin incisions. The knots are again tied subcutaneously.
  - ▲ The skin overlying the transabdominal fixation sutures should be released with a clamp to avoid dimpling of the skin (Figures 16-8 and 16-9).

Step 4. Postoperative Steps

- The orogastric tube and bladder catheter are removed in the operating room.
- Patients can be started on a regular diet after the operation, but if extensive bowel manipulation and adhesiolysis were done during the operation, the surgeon may prefer to keep the patient NPO with a nasogastric tube until bowel function returns.
- Antibiotics are continued for 24 hours, and heparin is continued until the patient is ambulatory unless the patient's comorbidities demand more prolonged therapy.
- For pain control, we favor narcotic patient controlled analgesia (PCA).
- We routinely place an abdominal binder for 1 month to help reduce seroma formation.
- Patients usually return to light duty within 1 week and resume full activity in 3 to 4 weeks.

Step 5. Pearls and Pitfalls

Patients with Defects Near the Costal Margin

Fixation at the superior edge of the mesh will be difficult in the upper abdomen, and patients should be counseled on a higher recurrence rate:

- Tacking to the diaphragm should be avoided because of the pain it will cause and the fact that it will likely only result in injury to the diaphragm without much enhancement of the mesh's fixation.
- Transfascial sutures will not be possible here and attempts to suture between the ribs should also be avoided as they may lead to pleural effusions.

The lack of fixation is supplanted by overlapping the hernia defect superiorly by more than the recommended 4 cm:

- To help achieve adequate coverage, the falciform ligament is divided up to the bare area of the liver.

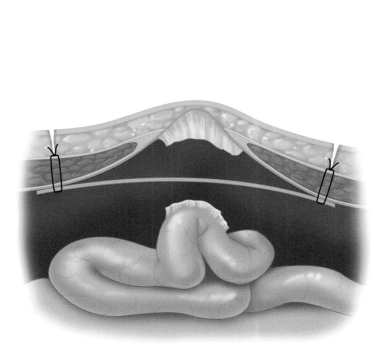

Figure 16-6

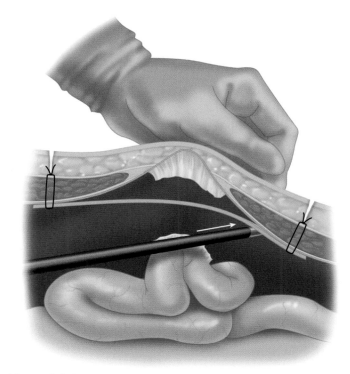

Figure 16-7

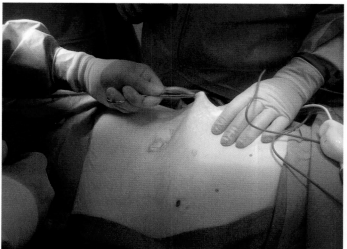

Figure 16-8

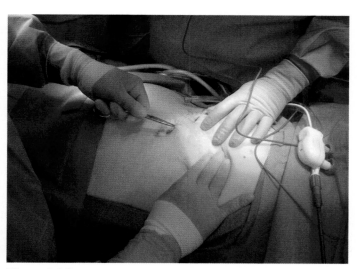

Figure 16-9

- The mesh is then placed between the liver and abdominal wall. It is fixated by tacking to the costal margin bony structures in as few areas as possible, with the goal of orienting the mesh to lie flat against the abdominal wall.
- Care should be taken to avoid injury to the infracostal neurovascular bundle.

Patients with Defects in the Pelvic Region

To achieve adequate caudal coverage of the hernia, we recommend several additional steps:
- First, we dissect the urinary bladder away from the anterior abdominal wall. To do this we place a three-way stopcock on the catheter to inflate and deflate the bladder. This will define the bladder and help avoid injury to the bladder (Figure 16-10).
- Once the bladder is dissected, it is retracted posteriorly and the pubic symphysis and Cooper's ligaments are identified. The inferior edge of the mesh is then placed in this retropubic space and can be secured to Cooper's ligaments laterally with nonabsorbable spiral tacks.
- In the midline, the mesh is sutured to the anterior abdominal wall using a transfascial technique or an intracorporeal technique if the surgeon doesn't feel a transfascial stitch is possible.

Intestinal Injury

If an injury is encountered during the course of the operation, then a staged approach is recommended.
- First the injury is repaired, the patient's abdomen is closed and the patient is allowed to recover.
- After a few weeks, the patient can be taken back to the operating room for placement of a permanent mesh.

Parastomal Hernia

A laparoscopic repair can still be done using the same principles of the Sugarbaker technique.
- The parastomal hernia is reduced, the stoma site is not moved, and the mesh is placed around the defect using the same goal of a 4-cm overlap.
- A lateral outlet is made for the intestine that leads to the ostomy.

Selected References

Turner PL, Park AE: *Laparoscopic repair of ventral incisional hernias: pros and cons.* Surg Clin of No Amer 88(1):85-100 2008.
Varghese TK, Wu A, Murayama K: *Ventral hernia repair.* In Jones DB, Wu J, Soper NJ (editors): Laparoscopic Surgery: Principles and Procedures ed 2. New York, Marcel Dekker, 2004, pp. 159-170.
Saber AA, Rao AJ, Itawi EA, et al: *Occult ventral hernia defects: a common finding during laparoscopic ventral hernia repair.* Am J Surg 195(4): 471-3 2008.
Scott D, Jones DB. *Hernias and abdominal wall defects.* In Norton JA, Bollinger RR, Chang AE, et al (editors): Surgery Scientific Basis and Current Practice. New York, Springer-Verlag, 2008, pp. 1133. 1178.

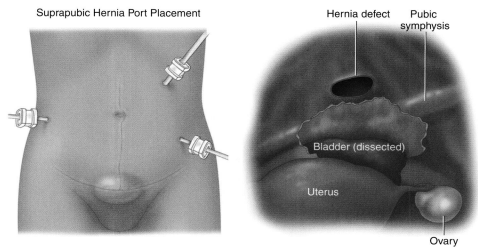

Suprapubic Hernia Port Placement

Hernia defect   Pubic symphysis

Bladder (dissected)

Uterus

Ovary

Figure 16-10

CHAPTER 17

ENDOSCOPIC COMPONENT SEPARATION

David Earle and Jessica Evans

Step 1. Surgical Anatomy

- The rectus abdominis muscle is a paired muscle running vertically from the costal margin to the inguinal ligament. It is separated in the midline by the linea alba. Along its lateral borders are the fused aponeuroses of the external oblique, internal oblique, and transversus abdominis muscles.
- Abdominal wall hernias often occur in the midline at the linea alba. Often, a great distance separates the rectus muscle bellies. During repair, there may be excessive tension when the muscles are pulled together to re-create the midline. One technique that can be helpful is to release the rectus abdominis muscle from some of its lateral attachments to pull it medially.
- To separate the rectus abdominis muscle from the external oblique muscle, an incision needs to be lateral to the fused aponeuroses of the external and internal oblique muscles. This will allow the internal oblique/transversus abdominis/rectus abdominis unit to "release" medially. Full separation of the flimsy fibroareolar connective tissue between the oblique muscles will maximize mobilization of the rectus muscle bellies medially (Figure 17-1).

Step 2. Preoperative Considerations

Patient Preparation

- Endoscopic component separation (ECS) is most useful for patients with midline defects of more than 5 to 8 cm in width as measured between the medial borders of the rectus muscle bellies (Figure 17-2).
- Symptoms associated with large defects that can be improved with component separation include a large abdominal wall deformity, difficulty leaning forward, difficulty fitting clothes, and discomfort related to pressure pushing the skin outward. Less clearly associated symptoms include inability to carry out activities of daily living or work, skin ulceration, and difficulties with an ostomy appliance if present.

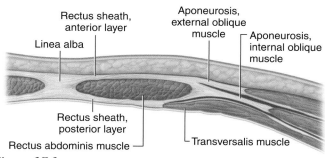

Figure 17-1

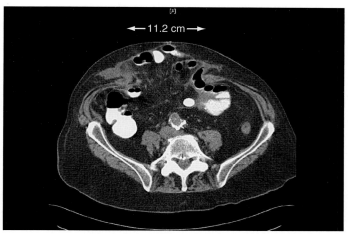

Figure 17-2

- Component separation can be incorporated with open, laparoscopic, or laparoscopic-assisted hernia repair. Patient selection for each approach is based on the specific clinical characteristics, most of which can be determined preoperatively with a physical examination and computed tomography (CT). Open and laparoscopic-assisted approaches have the advantage of suturing the midline together with more accuracy and strength, compared to laparoscopic techniques.
  - ▲ An *open* approach is typically planned for those requiring scar revision (because of ulcers, thin skin, previous skin graft, or unsightly scar) or explantation of a large prosthetic.
  - ▲ A *laparoscopic-assisted* approach is usually planned for those with defects wider than approximately 10 cm because of the difficulties of reapproximating the rectus abdominis muscle with percutaneous and laparoscopic techniques.
  - ▲ A full *laparoscopic* approach is usually planned for those with defects less than approximately 10 cm in width.
- Preoperative CT is useful for operative planning if considering a laparoscopic or laparoscopic-assisted approach. The exact dimensions of the defect can be ascertained, along with the calculated location of the lateral border of the rectus abdominis muscle. The latter measurement is particularly important if performing ECS as the initial portion of the operation (Figure 17-3).
- *Prior abdominal access* in the vicinity of the rectus and oblique muscles pose potential difficulty because of adhesions between fascial planes. Examples include open appendectomy or laterally based ostomy sites.

Equipment and Instrumentation

- A standard handheld Bovie is adequate for dissection of the space between the oblique muscles. Deep thin retractors such as S-retractors are also useful during this part of the procedure.
- A dissecting balloon (OMSPDB 1000 Covidien, Mansfield, Massachusetts) facilitates the creation of the space between the oblique muscles prior to insufflation (Figure 17-4).
- A port with a balloon at the distal end (OMST10BT Covidien, Mansfield, Massachusetts) or a valveless port (AirSeal; Surgiquest, Orange, CT) helps prevent leakage during insufflation. There is limited space between the muscles. This port can be pulled all the way back to the tip, and the balloon tip prevents inadvertent removal of the port. This gives the best view of the small space (Figure 17-5).

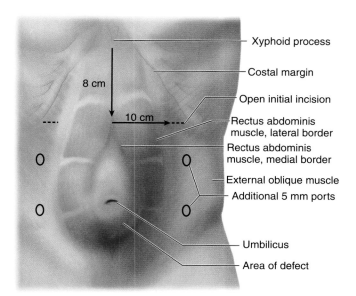

Xyphoid process

Costal margin

Open initial incision

Rectus abdominis
muscle, lateral border

Rectus abdominis
muscle, medial border

External oblique muscle

Additional 5 mm ports

Umbilicus

Area of defect

8 cm

10 cm

Figure 17-3

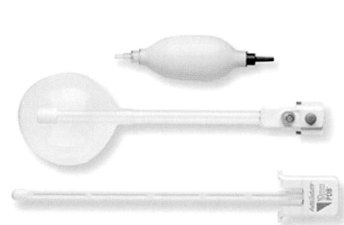

Figure 17-4

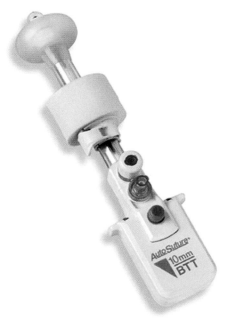

Figure 17-5

Anesthesia

- Regardless of the exact operative approach, general anesthesia is required. Consideration should also be given for epidural catheter placement to assist with postoperative pain management.
- Antibiotics: routine prophylactic antibiotics to cover gram-positive organisms should be administered prior to surgery. In longer cases, antibiotic redosing may be necessary. Postoperative antibiotics are not routinely required.
- A three-way bladder catheter is useful to avoid injury to the urinary bladder when dissecting in the pelvis. The bladder is filled with approximately 300 cc of saline and the catheter clamped. Once this portion of the dissection is complete, the clamp is removed.

Room Setup and Patient Positioning

- The patients are in the supine position, being sure to have the costal margins and lateral abdominal wall prepped in the area of the surgical field.
- Tucking both arms at the patient's sides is helpful for the laparoscopic approaches, as both the surgeon and assistant stand on the same side. This is particularly useful when working in the pelvis.
- A sterile adhesive drape is utilized to hold the drapes in place and prevent significant contact between the skin and prosthetic.

Step 3: Operative Steps

Port Placement and Creation of Plane beneath the External Oblique Muscle

- A 2- to 4-cm transverse incision is made inferior to the costal margin, approximately 3 cm lateral to the lateral border of the rectus abdominis muscle.
- Completely clean off and divide the thin anterior fascia overlying the external oblique muscle body, and definitively identify the correct orientation of its fibers (Figure 17-6).
- The muscle fibers are bluntly separated until the plane between the oblique muscles is confirmed and entered, taking care not to go too deep into or through the internal oblique. The internal oblique aponeurosis is smooth and whitish in color.

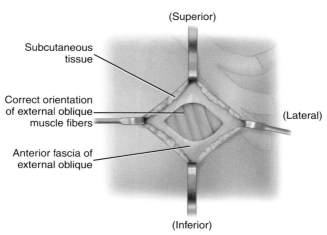

Figure 17-6

- While elevating and holding the external oblique muscle fibers apart with a small retractor, place the balloon dissector in this plane between the oblique muscles, and gently push the tip toward the inguinal ligament inferior to the level of the anterior superior iliac spine. The balloon dissector is serially inflated and deflated, each sequence pulling the balloon more cephalad. Two to three sequences are usually adequate to fully separate the muscles.
- The balloon is too large to separate the muscles medial and superior to the initial access incision. This portion of the dissection is easily accomplished with the surgeon's finger. Palpation of the costal margin also confirms the correct plane of dissection in this area.
- The balloon dissector is then removed, replaced with a balloon-tipped or AirSeal port, and the space between the oblique muscles insufflated with carbon dioxide. If the correct plane has been dissected, the initial inspection will reveal a cavity with external oblique anterior and internal oblique posterior, each with the normal orientation of their fibers. Both the medial and lateral aspects of the cavity will be fused together, and flimsy fibroareolar connective tissue is seen along these attachments. The medial boundary represents the lateral border of the rectus sheath.
- Two 5-mm transverse incisions are then made inferior to the initial access site, evenly spaced in the craniocaudad direction. The additional port sites should be lateral enough to allow for instrument and scope manipulation. The instrument used to divide the aponeurosis will be placed through the middle port, and the scope will be placed through the ports in the upper and lower quadrants.

Division of the External Oblique Aponeurosis

- Blunt dissection is performed to free up any remaining fibroareolar connective tissue and completely separate the internal and external oblique muscles.
- The division of the external oblique aponeurosis is usually associated with minimal bleeding as the plane is avascular. Laparoscopic Metzenbaum scissors are adequate in most circumstances except when nearby subcutaneous and muscular blood vessels are injured. We encourage the use of monopolar cautery to supplement the shears or a 5-mm energy source such as an ultrasonic coagulator if needed (Figure 17-7).
- The internal oblique/transversus abdominis/rectus abdominis unit will visibly "release" medially as the aponeurosis is divided. You should immediately see subcutaneous fat above the fascia (Figure 17-8).
- The aponeurotic division should begin almost directly medial to the middle port, approximately 5 to 10 mm lateral to the rectus-external oblique junction. The incision is continued vertically parallel to this junction all the way to the inguinal ligament inferiorly and above the costal margin superiorly. It is common to view and divide muscle fibers above the costal margin (Figure 17-9).
- Once the aponeurosis is divided, gentle dissection of the connective tissue in the subcutaneous space should be performed to gain significant additional mobility.
- The ports are then removed under direct vision, and the carbon dioxide is allowed to escape. No drain is left in place.

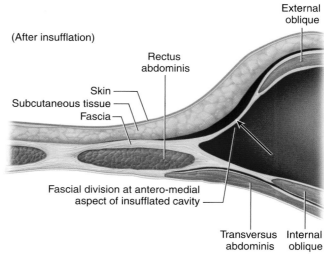

Figure 17-7

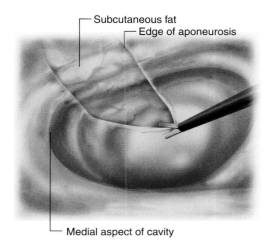

Figure 17-8

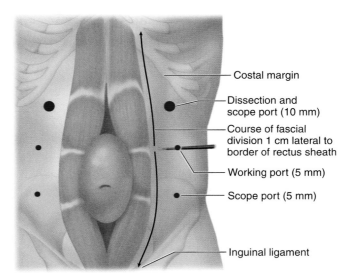

Figure 17-9

Port Closure

- Once the operation is complete, the anterior fascia of the external oblique is closed with absorbable suture.
- The skin is closed with subcuticular absorbable suture and adhesive skin closure strips.

Options for Hernia Repair

Bilateral endoscopic component separation (BECS) improves options for hernia repair, especially in complex abdominal wall reconstructions. There are few options when midline tissue is missing as in loss of domain or when the midline tissue needs to be excised as in infected mesh or with a takedown of an enterocutaneous fistula. BECS allows closure of the midline, which can be done in the following four ways:

- *Open hernia repair (laparotomy first).* Begin with laparotomy and adhesiolysis first in order to accurately define the medial border of the rectus muscle and determine if the midline can be closed without tension. If the midline cannot be brought together, then switch to BECS. Once adequate release is achieved, then finish with retromuscular prosthetic placement and closure of abdominal wall over prosthetic.
- *Open (BECS first).* A preoperative CT scan is critical to accurately identify the lateral border of the rectus. The lateral border is marked in the operating room by measurements acquired from CT scan and physical exam. Once the BECS is completed, then move to open laparotomy and adhesiolysis, retromuscular prosthetic placement, and closure of abdominal wall over prosthetic. This is usually necessary when the defect is greater than 10 to 12 cm in width and extends the full length of the previous midline incision. Despite the difficulty identifying lateral border of rectus abdominis muscles, this is the preferred approach because the laparotomy incision is open for less time compared to the sequence described in the first option (Figure 17-10).
- *Laparoscopic assisted.* Begin with laparoscopic adhesiolysis and identification of lateral border of rectus abdominis muscle, then proceed with BECS. Or BECS could be done first (using CT scan data to locate the lateral border of the rectus muscles) followed by laparoscopic adhesiolysis. Once the BECS, adhesiolysis, and measurement of the defect is complete, then create a small laparotomy in center of defect, pass the prosthetic through the midline incision/defect, and close the midline. The final step is laparoscopic fixation of prosthetic to cover the defect. It is critical to place the laparoscopic ports lateral to the anticipated edge of the prosthetic. This can be used for defects that are relatively small, between 5 and 12 cm, and do not extend the full length of the previous incision.
- *Totally laparoscopic.* Begin with laparoscopic adhesiolysis and identification of lateral border of rectus abdominis muscle, then proceed with BECS. The closure of the abdominal wall is done with percutaneous transfascial fixation sutures. The closure is reinforced with a retromuscular prosthetic placement and fixation. This allows for abdominal wall closure without an incision; rather a series of small incisions. This is generally better for narrow defects in the range of 5 to 8 cm in width that run the complete length of the old incision.

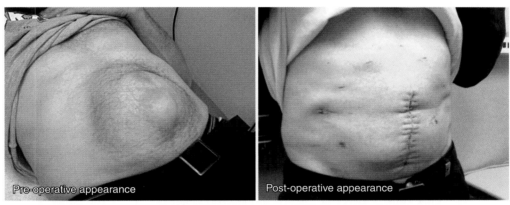

Figure 17-10

Step 4. Postoperative Care

- Overall postoperative care is the same as for hernia repair patients without component separation.
- If there is tension on the fascial closure, keeping the patient's trunk slightly flexed for the first 4 to 5 days helps to reduce this tension. The tissues should stretch to accommodate the tension within the first week.
- An abdominal wall binder is worn for the first few weeks postoperatively for patient comfort and to potentially prevent seroma formation in the space between the oblique muscles.

Step 5. Pearls and Pitfalls

- Locate the lateral border of the rectus abdominis muscle by manual palpation, laparoscopy, or CT measurements from known landmarks (such as midline and costal margin). Incorrectly identifying the lateral border of the rectus abdominis muscle will result in separation of the wrong muscle layers. Errors in identifying the lateral border of the rectus abdominis muscle usually occur because the surgeon has anticipated that this landmark is more medial than it actually is. In other words, it is often *more lateral than one would expect.*
- Missing the plane between external and internal oblique on initial open access usually occurs because the dissection was too deep. To rectify the situation, enlarge the incision slightly and move to a more lateral location on the external oblique. Slowly spread the external oblique muscle fibers with a blunt instrument to positively identify the whitish fascia or aponeurosis of the internal oblique.
- If the initial access incision is placed too close to either the costal margin or the lateral border of the rectus sheath, the balloon-tipped port will interfere with division of the external oblique aponeurosis. Partial deflation of the balloon can give additional room to assist in this situation. Use of the AirSeal port eliminates this problem.
- Using an energy source too close to a balloon-tipped port can break the balloon. Evacuate some of the air from the balloon, and have the assistant hold the tip of the port lateral to help avoid this problem.
- Lateral abdominal port sites can be shared for both the laparoscopic portion of the procedure and the ECS. If the initial access site for the ECS was also used for an intraperitoneal port, extra care must be taken to ensure that the correct plane for dissection is accessed. Gas may escape into the peritoneal cavity during ECS. All port sites used for intraperitoneal laparoscopy that traverse the component separation should be closed to avoid port site hernia.
- If the defect cannot be closed completely, leave the middle portion open. This will be determined by the tension experienced during closure. The remaining defect will be significantly smaller than the original defect, and it will be covered by the prosthetic. Flexing the patient's trunk during closure can alleviate some tension.
- Patients with significant loss of domain may exhibit abdominal compartment syndrome with midline fascial closure, even after completion of component separation. This is unusual, but the surgeon should ask the anesthesia staff about airway pressures during and after closure of large defects or those associated with massive hernia sacs.

Selected References

Lowe JB, Garza JR, et al: Endoscopically assisted "components separation" for closure of abdominal wall defects. *Plast Reconstr Surg*: 105(2), 720-9; quiz 730, 2000.
Ramirez OM, Ruas E, Dellon AL: "Components separation" method for closure of abdominal-wall defects: an anatomic and clinical study. *Plast Reconstr Surg*: 86(3): 519-26, 1990.
Rosen MJ, Jin J, et al: Laparoscopic component separation in the single-stage treatment of infected abdominal wall prosthetic removal. Hernia: 11(5): 435-40, 2007.

18

PERITONEAL DIALYSIS CATHETER PLACEMENT

William P. Robinson III and Matthew T. Menard

Step 1. Surgical Anatomy

- The peritoneal dialysis (PD) catheter should enter the abdomen through the rectus muscle medial to the epigastric vessels, with the inner cuff positioned at the level of the parietal peritoneum.
- The PD catheter should exit the skin lateral to the abdominal entrance site, with the external cuff positioned approximately 2 cm from the exit site in a subcutaneous tunnel.
- The sites for catheter placement should be evaluated in the supine and sitting positions and in relation to undergarments to ensure that the patient can easily access the catheter. Placement below the belt line, within a skin fold, or in a location where body habitus and clothing cause catheter kinking or rubbing should be avoided.
- Previous abdominal incisions are not a contraindication to the laparoscopic approach but may direct the safest location for port placement.
- The course of the epigastric arteries must be visualized during port insertion through the rectus abdominis.

Step 2. Preoperative Considerations

- The indications for laparoscopic PD catheter placement are identical to those of PD catheter placement via conventional minilaparotomy, blind percutaneous Seldinger, or peritoneoscopic technique. Indications include an inability to tolerate hemodialysis (e.g., heart disease or extensive vascular disease) or a stated preference for peritoneal dialysis. The benefit of peritoneal dialysis is the ability to perform dialysis at home as long as the patient or an assistant has the capacity to perform exchanges properly.
- Laparoscopic PD catheter placement allows complete visualization of precise intra-abdominal implantation, the ability to perform adhesiolysis if required, and the ability to secure the catheter in the pelvis if desired. For these reasons, both surgeons and nephrologists increasingly prefer laparoscopic PD catheter placement in comparison to the older methods of percutaneous Seldinger technique, peritoneoscopic approach, and open placement via minilaparotomy.

- Contraindications to PD include the extensive adhesions that would prohibit adequate dialysate flow, an irreparable abdominal wall hernia, diaphragmatic defects predisposing to hydrothorax, and severe lung disease to a degree that increased intra-abdominal volume would compromise respiratory function. Morbid obesity is a relative contraindication.
- Most experts feel that the initial higher cost of laparoscopic PD catheter placement is more than offset by the lower incidence of costly later complications in comparison with open surgical placement or blind percutaneous placement.
- Appropriate preoperative teaching and arrangements for initial supervised sterile dressing changes should be made before operation.

Patient Preparation and Anesthesia

- Patients wash their abdomen with chlorhexidine the evening prior to surgery.
- In the setting of known constipation, an enema or suppository can be given preoperatively to facilitate rectosigmoid emptying.
- Hair is removed with electric clippers.
- Patients who continue to make urine empty their bladder immediately before operation or have a Foley catheter inserted.
- One to 2 grams of cefazolin IV is given 30 minutes before the operation.
- The patient is placed supine on a bed capable of Trendelenburg positioning.
- General anesthesia is employed.

Step 3: Operative Steps

- The operative goals of PD catheter placement, all of which maximize function and prevent complications, include placement of the catheter tip deep in the dependent portion of the pelvis, appropriate positioning of the dual felt cuffs and subcutaneous portion of the catheter, and creation of a functional exit site.
- Multiple laparoscopic PD catheter placement techniques have been described, using a range of 1 to 3 laparoscopic ports. All techniques that allow for placement under continuous direct vision, including descriptions of a "1-port" approach, require at least 2 fascial defects. Although some surgeons call their technique "one-port", they use one port for a camera and then another hole is made in the abdominal wall to insert the catheter without placing an actual laparoscopic trocar.
- Conventional minilaparotomy should be considered in patients with severe cardiopulmonary disease who may not tolerate pneumoperitoneum.
- The abdomen is widely prepped from the xiphoid to the pubis, allowing for the possibility of a midline laparotomy.

Two-Port Technique

Access and Port Placement

- Incision locations are marked on the patient after placing the PD catheter in the desired location on the abdomen as a guide. With the distal catheter coil overlying the superior pubis, the eventual location of the deep cuff is marked on the skin. This point corresponds to the anticipated trocar entry point through the fascia into the peritoneum.
- A 5-mm curvilinear incision is made just below the umbilicus, and the subcutaneous tissue is spread bluntly. If previous periumbilical or midline incisions are present, this initial port placement can be made lateral to the rectus muscle near the level of the umbilicus. In patients who have had previous extensive abdominal surgery, placement of the initial trocar is best performed with a cutdown under direct vision.

- With upward traction on the abdominal wall, a Veress needle is placed via this incision through the midline fascia. The intraperitoneal position is confirmed with a hanging drop test and low-pressure readings on initiation of insufflation. The peritoneal cavity is then insufflated to 15 mmHg with carbon dioxide (Figure 18-1).
- A 5-mm trocar is placed into the abdomen through the infraumbilical incision, through which a 5-mm 30-degree laparoscopic camera is placed.
- Diagnostic laparoscopy is undertaken with attention directed to identifying any inguinal or abdominal wall hernias requiring prophylactic repair or adhesions or omental redundancy that could potentially obstruct pelvic placement or catheter drainage.
- In the event that adhesiolysis, omentectomy, or tacking up of redundant omentum proves necessary to allow pelvic placement of the catheter, a third 5- to 10-mm working port is placed through the contralateral abdominal wall.
- A second 8-mm horizontal stab incision is made 4 to 5 cm lateral and 2 to 3 cm inferior to the umbilicus. An 8-mm nonbladed trocar (Ethicon Excel B8LT; Ethicon, Somerville, New Jersey) is advanced subcutaneously in a medial and slightly caudal trajectory toward the pelvis. A 5- to 6-cm subcutaneous tunnel is created before angling the trocar perpendicular to the abdominal wall and piercing the intervening fascia and peritoneal envelope. Care should be taken to direct the trocar through the rectus abdominis muscle medial to the epigastric vessel, which can often be visualized with the laparoscope. All intraperitoneal manipulations should be done under direct vision.

Equipment description

Introduction of Peritoneal Dialysis Catheter

- A 62-cm curled-tip peritoneal dialysis catheter with two felt cuffs (Kendall Quinton Curl Cath, Covidien, Mansfield, Massachusetts) is inserted into the 8-mm trocar with the aid of a flexible Bard ureteral stylet and directed to the pelvis under direct camera vision. It should be noted that a 7- to 8-mm trocar must be used, as the Dacron cuffs of the PD catheter will not pass through a trocar smaller than 7 mm (Figure 18-2).
- Once the catheter is intraperitoneal, the stylet is withdrawn approximately 4 to 5 cm to allow the curled atraumatic catheter tip to form, and the catheter is directed deep into the retrovesicle space. The stylet is slowly removed while ensuring the curved tip remains in the desired location.

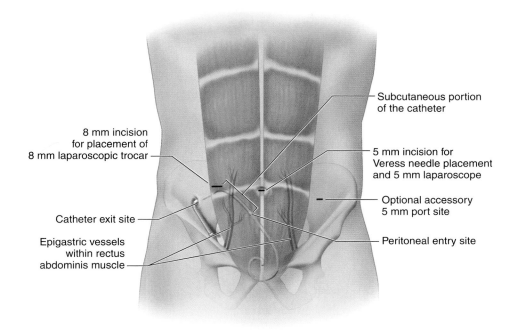

8 mm incision
for placement of
8 mm laparoscopic trocar

Subcutaneous portion
of the catheter

5 mm incision for
Veress needle placement
and 5 mm laparoscope

Catheter exit site

Optional accessory
5 mm port site

Epigastric vessels
within rectus
abdominis muscle

Peritoneal entry site

Figure 18-1

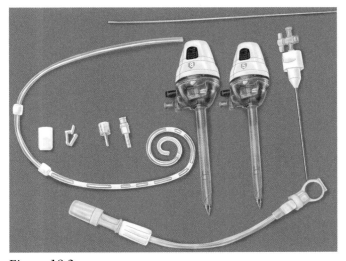

Figure 18-2

- The catheter is then positioned such that the inner cuff lies just exterior to the level of the parietal peritoneum so the optimal scarring in of the catheter can take place. The catheter is secured by hand externally, and the trocar is then carefully removed over the catheter, while ensuring that the inner cuff remains in position and the outer cuff lies fully within the subcutaneous tunnel (Figure 18-3).
- The catheter exit site should allow the catheter to point medially as it exits the skin and serves to further separate the external cuff from the exit site.

Subcutaneous Tunnel

- A small stab incision the width of the catheter is made slightly inferior and lateral to the 8-mm external wound. A tonsil clamp is advanced to create a short arcing tunnel, and the end of the catheter is grasped and brought out of the skin incision. No securing suture is used at this site. Alternatively, a Faller stylet can be attached to the end of the catheter and directed from lateral incision through the new exit site.

Completion of Procedure

- Catheter function is tested by injection of 60 cc and aspiration of 30 to 40 cc of heparinized Normal Saline (1000 U/L).
- Proper positioning of the catheter is confirmed with the camera before trocar removal and desufflation of the abdomen (Figure 18-4).
- A sterile extension to the PD catheter is attached if available. The fascial defects do not require closure. The two skin incisions are closed with a 4-0 subcuticular Monocryl suture and Steri-Strips. Sterile adhesive dressings are applied.

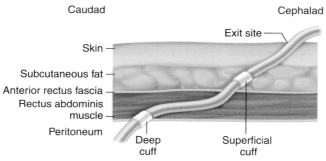

Figure 18-3

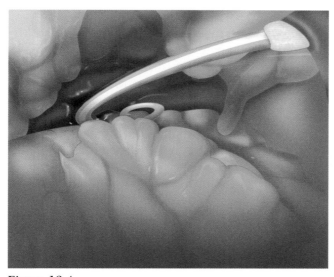

Figure 18-4

Laparoscopic-Guided Technique with Quinton Percutaneous Insertion Kit

- Intraperitoneal insufflation and camera access is obtained as described earlier.
- A Quinton percutaneous insertion kit (Tyco Healthcare Group LP, Mansfield, Massachusetts) is used for catheter placement through the rectus muscle in a paramedian location infero-lateral to the umbilicus. The kit allows placement of a 16 Fr Pull-Apart introducer sheath via Seldinger technique. A Swan Neck Curl-Cath double-cuffed PD catheter (Kendall Quinton Curl Cath, Tyco Healthcare Corp., REF 8888413401) is advanced through the sheath to the desired location. The leaves of the sheath are then pulled apart, leaving the catheter in place.
- Some authors utilizing this technique have described placement of an additional contralateral 2- to 5-mm port to allow use of a grasper to direct the PD catheter into the pelvis. Others have advocated use of a percutaneously placed permanent nylon loop on the peritoneal surface of the ipsilateral pelvic wall. The catheter is fed through the sheath as a means of pelvic fixation.
- An inferolateral exit site is fashioned with a stab incision and subcutaneous tunneling as described previously.

Presternal Catheter Placement

- Utilization of a Swan Neck Presternal Catheter (Covidien, Mansfield, Massachusetts), a 112.8-cm catheter with an intraperitoneal component coupled to a long subcutaneous thoracic segment, has been described for patients in whom an abdominal exit site is not suitable because of body habitus, stomas, incontinence, or a preference for baths rather than showers. Intraperitoneal catheter placement is carried out laparoscopically as described earlier, though the catheter is introduced through the rectus muscle above the level of the umbilicus. The thoracic portion of the tubing is connected via a titanium connector to the abdominal component. A 2- to 3-cm parasternal incision is made at the level of the second interspace, and a subcutaneous pocket is created to accommodate the arced section of the thoracic segment, which allows the catheter to exit pointing inferiorly. The thoracic component is tunneled subcutaneously to this incision. Finally, the catheter is tunneled to the exit site stab wound several centimeters inferior to the parasternal incision. This technique is associated with low rates of infection and excellent overall long-term function.

Step 4. Postoperative Care

- Ideally, the catheter should be secured in a stable position and not used for 4 to 6 weeks in order to allow scarring of the fascial defects and healing of the subcutaneous tunnel. A minimum of 2 weeks should be allowed from placement until use, because there is a higher incidence of catheter leakage when used within 2 weeks of placement.

- Sterile dressing changes should not occur more than once per week for 2 weeks. Gentle daily exit site cleansing can begin at 2 weeks, and showering can begin at 1 month if healing has been good. Use of sharp objects such as safety pins or scissors should be avoided around the catheter.
- Patients should avoid heavy physical activity including straining. Patients should wear loose-fitting clothing so that pressure is not placed on the catheter site.
- Patients should promptly report any systemic or local symptoms or signs of infection including pain, redness, or excessive drainage at surgical sites.

Step 5. Pearls and Pitfalls

Infectious Complications

- Exit-site infection is signaled by purulent or bloody drainage around the catheter. It leads to peritonitis in 25% to 50% of patients. Culture-specific antibiotic therapy should be instituted for 2 to 6 weeks. Failure of medical therapy generally indicates cuff or tunnel infection and requires catheter removal. Tunnel infection is signaled by erythema, tenderness, or swelling over the subcutaneous catheter tunnel. Catheters can infrequently be salvaged by debridement of the infectious focus. However, catheter removal with either replacement through clean tissue planes (if there is no evidence of peritonitis) or delayed replacement after interval antibiotic treatment is almost always required.
- Peritonitis is the most common infectious complication of PD access. Peritonitis refractory to antibiotics or associated with a tunnel infection is an indication for catheter removal. Severe or recurrent infection often prompts transfer from peritoneal dialysis to hemodialysis.

Noninfectious Complications

- Early leakage (<30 days), indicated by dialysate in the subcutaneous tissues, is caused by failure of the peritoneum to close around the catheter or at port sites. Treatment includes cessation of PD for 1 to 2 weeks and prophylactic antibiotics. Exploration of the catheter entry site into the abdomen or port sites and repair of the tissues around the cuff are required if conservative treatments fails.
- Late leakage (>30 days) of dialysate into the subcutaneous tissues often manifests as edema of the abdominal wall or drainage problems during dialysis. Open or laparoscopic exploration and repair of suspected leak sites are required.
- Catheter displacement complicates 2% to 30% of cases. It is manifest by flow dysfunction and poor catheter drainage. Migration out of the pelvis can also lead to pain caused by peritoneal irritation.

- Catheter obstruction may result in both inflow and outflow problems or isolated outflow failure. Obstruction of inflow and outflow is usually caused by clot or fibrin ingrowth into the catheter side holes. Thrombolysis can be attempted, but catheter replacement is often required. Outflow difficulty can be secondary to migration from the pelvis but also can be the result of adherent adjacent omentum or bowel acting as a one-way valve. Laparoscopic repositioning is often successful in this instance.
- Pericannular leaks and hernias complicate 1% to 27% of procedures.
- Superficial cuff extrusion is usually seen when the cuff is placed too close to the lateral incision. Alternatively, if the catheter is tunneled subcutaneously in such a way that the catheter is under tension, the memory of the tubing will cause the catheter to extrude outwardly over time, potentially causing exposure of the cuff.
- Hernias, which result from the increased intra-abdominal pressure generated by the dialysate infusion, are seen in 10% to 25% of patients on PD. Some of these occur at laparoscopic port sites. For this reason, trocar size should be the smallest possible to accommodate the PD catheter, camera, and additional instruments for adhesiolysis as required.
- Preoperative planning of the incisions and the exit site is crucial to successful catheter placement.
- Proper selection of trocars and instrumentation allows one to minimize the size of fascial defects and the risk of hernia formation without compromising laparoscopic visualization.
- Appropriate placement of both inner and outer cuffs and optimal tunneling is critical to durable catheter function and minimizes catheter complications.

Selected References

Carrillo SA, Ghersi MM, Unger SW: Laparoscopic-assisted peritoneal dialysis catheter placement: a microinvasive technique. *Surg Endosc* 21(5):825-29, 2007.

Crabtree JH, Fishman A: A laparoscopic method for optimal peritoneal dialysis access. *Am Surg* 71(2):135-43, 2005.

Haggerty SP, Zeni TM, Carder M, et al: Laparoscopic peritoneal dialysis catheter insertion using a Quinton percutaneous insertion kit. *JSLS* 11(2):208-14, 2007.

Harissis HV, Katsios CS, Koliousi EL, et al: A new simplified one port laparoscopic technique of peritoneal dialysis catheter placement with intra-abdominal fixation. *Am J Surg* 192(1):125-29, 2006.

Schmidt SC, Pohle C, Langrehr JM, et al: Laparoscopic-assisted placement of peritoneal dialysis catheters: implantation technique and results. *J Laparoendosc Adv Surg Tech A* 17(5):596-99, 2007.

Twardowski ZJ: Peritoneal access: the past, present, and the future. *Contrib Nephrol* 150:195-201, 2006.

Twardowski ZJ, Prowant BF, Nichols WK, et al: Six-year experience with Swan neck presternal peritoneal dialysis catheter. *Perit Dial Int* 18(6):598-602, 1998.

IV

Lower Gastrointestinal Surgery

19

APPENDECTOMY

James P. Dolan

Step 1. Surgical Anatomy

- The appendix is a finger-like evagination of the proximal wall of the cecum. There has been extensive debate as to its evolutionary significance, with many considering it a vestigial organ in humans. More recent thought suggests an immune regulatory role involving immune-mediated maintenance of the normal gut flora.
- The appendix is about 10 cm long and 8 mm wide and has a luminal diameter of 1 to 3 mm. The three taenia coli merge at its base. Its sole blood supply is from the appendiceal artery, which originates as a branch of the ileocecal artery. The artery runs in the mesoappendix, the mesentery attaching the organ to the wall of the cecum. The position of the appendix can vary considerably and may be retrocecal in up to 65% of adults. The terminal ileum is an adjacent anatomic landmark.
- Because of its position in the right lower quadrant, pain in this area is usually suspicious for appendicitis. Variations in anatomic location, because of such conditions as advanced pregnancy or intestinal malrotation, are infrequent but should be suspected in the appropriate clinical context.

Step 2. Preoperative Consideration

Patient Preparation

- Appendicitis is the usual diagnosis prompting appendectomy.
- Although the diagnosis has classically been based on symptoms, physical exam, and laboratory results, there is increasing use of contrast-enhanced computed tomography (CT) in making the diagnosis.
- After the diagnosis is made, each patient should receive intravenous fluid hydration, intravenous broad-spectrum antibiotic suitable to cover enteric organisms, and intravenous analgesics.

- Patients should be consented for appendectomy and both laparoscopic and open approaches should be discussed with the patient, as well as the usual complications including bleeding, infection, and damage to intra-abdominal structures.
- Expedient operation is advised, although the urgency of the operation is usually dictated by patient symptoms, laboratory results, availability of the operating room or anesthesia resources, and results of imaging studies.
- Having consumed nothing by mouth within the preceding 6 hours is usually ideal from an anesthesia standpoint but is not an absolute contraindication to proceeding with the operation.

Equipment and Instrumentation

- Laparoscopic appendectomy is carried out using standard laparoscopic instruments, including atraumatic graspers and a hook electrocautery.
- A 5-mm or 10-mm, 30-degree or 45-degree laparoscope can be utilized. We usually use a 5-mm, 30-degree laparoscope for the procedure.
- Additional equipment includes the following:
  - ▲ Laparoscopic suction irrigator.
  - ▲ Specimen retrieval bag.
  - ▲ Endo GIA (Covidien Autosuture, Mansfield, Massachusetts) roticulating stapler with vascular (2.5 mm staple height) and gastrointestinal (3.5 mm staple height) cartridge loads; 45-mm cartridges are usually adequate and are easier to manipulate within the abdominal cavity than the 60-mm cartridges. Current versions of these staplers include a "lavender" (gastrointestinal) and "gold" (vascular) variant. These newer cartridges have changing staple heights along the length of the cartridge.

▲ The 10-mm laparoscopic clip applier should also be available in case there is a need to control a bleeding vessel or reinforce the staple line after deployment of the stapler.

▲ A pre-tied loop (Endoloop, Ethicon, Somerville, New Jersey) and a 10-mm laparoscopic clip applier are alternative options for controlling the appendiceal stump and artery if a stapler is not available.

▲ For cases in which there is severe suppuration, gangrene, or perforation, we usually place a 10-mm Blake Silicone Drain (Ethicon, Somerville, New Jersey) into the pelvis to remove postoperative fluid collections. It can be removed when drainage decreases to minimal amounts.

Anesthesia

◆ General anesthesia is required.

◆ Placement of an orogastric (OG) tube will facilitate decompression of the stomach if there is evidence of significant gastric content based on recent oral intake or evidence from computed tomography (CT) scan.

◆ If antibiotics have not already been administered, this should be done prior to incision in the operating room.

◆ A Foley catheter is required in order to decompress the bladder and decrease the risk of bladder injury. In uncircumcised males, make sure to pull the foreskin back over the glans penis after inserting the catheter.

Room Setup and Positioning

- The patient is positioned supine on the operating table.
- After general anesthesia is induced and the preceding steps have been performed, the patient's left arm should be safely tucked and padded. The right arm may be left "out" for anesthesia access.
- Ensure that the patient is secure on the table by testing in Trendelenburg and left-to-right roll positions.
- The operating surgeon is positioned on the patient's left side to the right of the scrub nurse or technician (Figure 19-1).
- The assistant is positioned on the patient's right side.
- The main display monitor is positioned off the patient's right leg directly in line with the appendix and operating surgeon's line of sight. If an additional display monitor is available, it should be positioned off the patient's left leg in line with the assistant surgeon. An additional monitor will reduce the assistant's neck strain but may increase difficulty in using the laparoscope because of the viewing angle and fulcrum effect.

Step 3. Operative Steps

Access and Port Placement

- The operating ports are a 12-mm and 5-mm port. The camera port can be 5 mm or 10 mm.
- The camera port is placed on the superior border of the umbilicus. Either a Veress needle or the Hassan technique may be used to gain access to the abdominal cavity.
- After establishing access, the abdomen is insufflated with carbon dioxide gas to 12 to 15 mmHg.
- A cursory laparoscopic examination is performed prior to subsequent port placement to assure the surgeon that there are no immediate contraindications to proceeding.
- There are a number of positions for the working ports of a laparoscopic appendectomy. We favor a 3-port (1 camera and 2 working) configuration with 2 variations:
  - ▲ Our favored variation effectively hides the 12-mm incision low on the abdomen, just above the pubic symphysis. It is used when cosmesis is an important consideration and in cases of uncomplicated appendicitis. (Figure 19-2a).

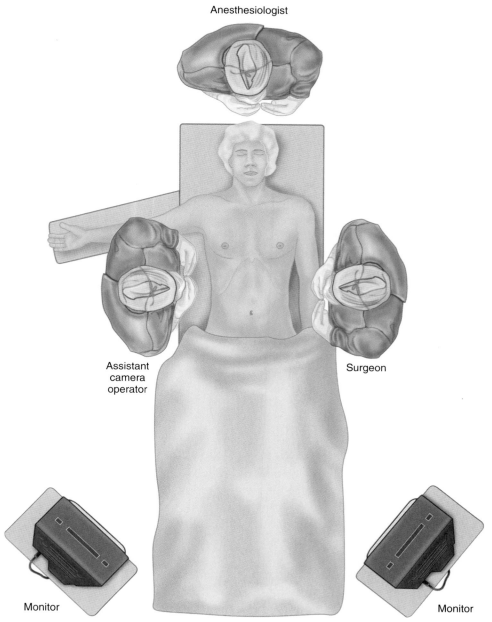

Figure 19-1

▲ Place the umbilical 5-mm camera port first.

▲ With the camera port established, a 5-mm right upper quadrant (RUQ) working port is placed under direct vision. An atraumatic grasper is introduced through this working port and used to guide placement of the final lower midline port.

▲ The incision should be 1 finger breadth above the superior border of the symphysis in order to avoid injury to the dome of the bladder.

▲ The peritoneum on the lower part of the abdomen tends to have some laxity and can "tent" inward during placement of the larger port. This is minimized by holding tissue up with the open jaws of the atraumatic grasper.

▲ Our second variation is used in pregnant patients and in cases where there is evidence of a significant left lower quadrant or lower abdominal inflammatory reaction in response to appendiceal infection.

▲ Here, to avoid a suprapubic port, we place the 12-mm port in the RUQ and a 5-mm port in the left lower quadrant (LLQ). This configuration may also provide a more comfortable range of motion if a stapler is being used to transect the appendix and mesoappendix (Figure 19-2b).

◆ Remember that the laparoscope can be moved to either of the working ports to facilitate better exposure of the appendix or to better assist the surgeon.

◆ There are now published reports of early experience with appendectomy using single incision laparoscopic surgery (SILS), particularly in the pediatric population, as well as natural orifice transluminal endoscopic surgery (NOTES).

Procedural Steps

Identification of the Appendix

◆ After camera and working port access has been established, the patient should be placed in 15- to 30-degree Trendelenburg position and rolled a similar extent to the patient's left. This will allow for better visualization of the right lower quadrant (RLQ).

◆ Identify anatomic landmarks (pelvic brim, right colon, sigmoid colon) to assist in recognizing the overall abdomen and help confirm the source of pathology.

◆ Begin by grasping normal-appearing small bowel and retracting it toward the left upper abdomen.

◆ Large blind sweep of bowel is discouraged, as this increases the risk of a hollow viscus injury or breaking open and spreading infection from an infected fluid collection. Bowel may also need to be removed from the pelvis, and loops may also be adhered to areas of local inflammation and infection in the RLQ.

◆ If possible, use a laparoscopic suction irrigator in one hand and an atraumatic grasper in the other, and suction reactive ascites or purulence as it is encountered. In addition to making it easier to visualize the operative field, this action will also remove infected fluid that might potentially spread and provide a focus for future abscess formation.

◆ At this point, significant appendicitis, if present, should not be difficult to visualize if the appendix originates from the anterior or inferior wall of the cecum or if there is a perforation (Figure 19-3).

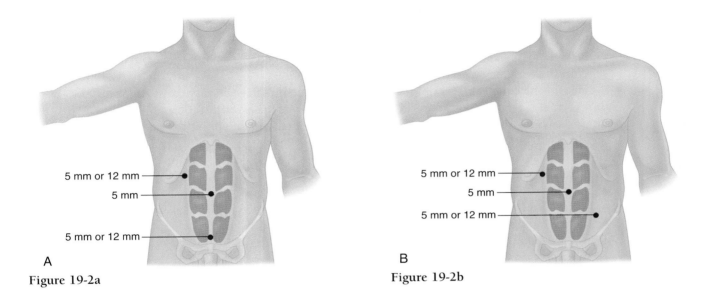

5 mm or 12 mm

5 mm

5 mm or 12 mm

A

Figure 19-2a

5 mm or 12 mm

5 mm

5 mm or 12 mm

B

Figure 19-2b

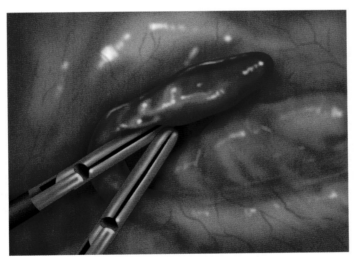

Figure 19-3

- The appendix may be difficult to visualize if it is retrocecal or if there is early infection that produces a minimal local inflammatory reaction. Locating and following one of the three taenia coli may help in locating the appendix, as these merge at its base.
- Often, complete visualization of the appendix will require two additional maneuvers:
  ▲ Division of the cecal fascia fused to the abdominal wall in the LLQ. This will allow for inferior and lateral to medial mobilization of the cecum in order to better locate a retrocecal appendix.
  ▲ Avoid extensive lateral to medial dissection of the cecum, as this brings one into the area of the iliac vessels and right ureter.
  ▲ Identification of the terminal ileum. This will allow identification of the ileocecal ligament (fold of Treves), which can be grasped, elevated, and manipulated to better locate or characterize the pathologic anatomy of the appendix. Rigorous retraction or manipulation of an inflamed terminal ileum may result in bowel injury (Figure 19-4).
- Because of the extent or stage of the disease, the appendix may be easy to locate or may be unrecognized against a background of inflammation, necrosis, or infection.
- Be prepared for significant tissue friability and bleeding, which will hinder visualization of the diseased appendix.
- Have suitable equipment available to allow safe completion of the procedure:
  ▲ Laparoscopic suction irrigator
  ▲ Surgical staplers and reloads
  ▲ Maxon or equivalent Endoloop
  ▲ 10-mm laparoscopic clip applier
  ▲ Surgical drains: Blake or Penrose brand closed suction drains
  ▲ Suture material for extracorporeal or extracorporeal suturing if needed. Polyglycolic acid sutures are favored over permanent material, which may provide a nidus for continued infection.

Division of the Appendiceal Stump

- For early appendicitis, a window is first created in the mesoappendix. The appendiceal artery is controlled by placement of a series of 10-mm Endo clips and is then transected. An Endo GIA vascular stapler load may also be used for controlling and transecting the artery. The appendix is removed after placing double Endoloops at its base or transecting it with an Endo GIA gastrointestinal stapler load.
- Organs with more advanced inflammation (serositis, global edema, suppuration, or gangrene without perforation) should have the mesoappendix controlled with a surgical staple load if possible, because the inflammation and edema may make it difficult to easily locate the appendiceal artery for clipping. Likewise, the appendiceal stump may be severely damaged down to its base and may require stapling onto the cecum:
  ▲ Partial cecectomy, if performed because of inflammation or infection of the base of appendix, is generally tolerated without clinical sequelae.
  ▲ Carefully inspect the mesoappendix staple line for bleeding. Use laparoscopic clips as needed for control of bleeding. The use of electrocautery may increase the risk of injury to bowel, colon, iliac vessels, or ureter.
- The appendix should be grasped by noninflamed tissue if possible to avoid perforation and possible soilage of the abdominal cavity. Other options include use of an Endoloop on the appendix or partial transection (using stapler or Endoloop) at viable tissue and removal of the diseases—usually distal portion—in an Endo Catch bag or other retrieval device.

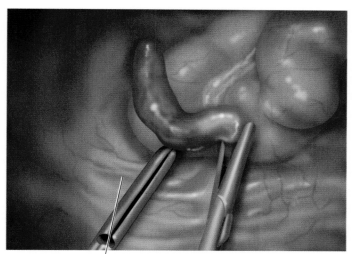

White line of Toldt

Figure 19-4

- In instances where there is considerable inflammation, appendiceal perforation with local containment, abscess, or complete degeneration of the appendix itself *without fecal contamination*, it is usually wise to avoid extensive manipulation of the cecum or widespread dissection in order to attempt to visualize innate anatomy. This may result in damage to small bowel or cecal perforation and convert a locally controlled infection into gross soilage of the abdominal cavity.
  - ▲ Instead, gently irrigate and aspirate the area and remove dead tissue as it presents itself.
  - ▲ Do not attempt to identify the "stump" if it is not clear to you where it might be.
  - ▲ Leave a pelvic surgical drain in place, and consider an additional drain in the area of the right colonic gutter if extensive irrigation, aspiration, and debris removal has been conducted.
- In instances where there is complete degeneration of the appendix itself *with fecal contamination*, it is usually wise to convert to an open procedure by means of a lower midline laparotomy. In these instances, it has been our experience that even advanced laparoscopic skills cannot assure a safe tissue repair and good local infection control.

Specimen Removal

- The appendix (intact or in pieces) is placed into a retrieval bag and removed through the 12-mm trocar.
- Finish by copiously irrigating the RLQ and pelvis and aspirating off as much irrigant as possible.

Closure

- Observe the surgical site under reduced pneumoperitoneum (6 to 10 mmHg) to check for bleeding prior to desufflating the abdomen and closure.
- Close the fascia of the 12-mm port site if technically possible. Skin incisions may be closed with tissue adhesive, absorbable subcuticular suture, or surgical staples.

Step 4. Postoperative Care

- The patient can be typically cared for on the regular surgical ward with intravenous fluids and pain medications.
- The orogastric tube and Foley catheter can be removed at the end of the operation.
- Intravenous (IV) antibiotics may be continued for 24 to 72 hours after operation in cases of acute, suppurative, necrotic, or perforated appendicitis.
- Early appendicitis may only require perioperative IV antibiotic use.
- Clear liquids can be initiated as tolerated. Patients are encouraged to ambulate and use incentive spirometry as early as possible to prevent DVT and atelectasis.

- ◆ Infectious complications related to the procedure range from 2% to 6% and include the following:
  - ▲ Wound infection
  - ▲ Intra-abdominal abscess
  - ▲ Enteritis or colitis
  - ▲ Pneumonia
  - ▲ Urinary tract infection
  - ▲ Liver abscess
- ◆ Other complications occur, on average, up to 2% of the time and include the following:
  - ▲ Bowel obstruction
  - ▲ Bowel perforation
  - ▲ Postoperative ileus
  - ▲ Bleeding (intra-abdominal or wound)
  - ▲ Bladder perforation
  - ▲ Urinary retention
  - ▲ Deep venous thrombosis
- ◆ Patients may return to full activity when they no longer require pain medication. This is usually between 1 and 7 days after surgery. Persistence of lower abdominal pain; episodes of diarrhea, dysuria, or urinary frequency; low-grade fevers; or persistent malaise should raise the suspicion of intra-abdominal abscess or some other infection or complication.

Step 5. Pearls and Pitfalls

- ◆ Either a Veress needle or the Hassan technique may be used to gain access to the abdominal cavity. The Hassan technique allows for a more controlled access but is not without complication itself.
- ◆ If an Endo GIA stapler was used to control the appendiceal artery, inspect the transected staple line very carefully under reduced intra-abdominal pressure to check for bleeding. Significant edema or inflammation of the mesoappendix as a result of adjacent appendicitis can predispose to suboptimal stapler performance and subsequent staple line bleeding.
- ◆ Always have a laparoscopic clip applier available in case there is the need to control bleeding from the appendiceal artery.
- ◆ The transected finger of a surgical glove may also be used to retrieve the appendix from the abdomen after transection. This mode of extraction is best suited for specimens with early appendicitis.
- ◆ A Foley catheter is mandatory for all cases to minimize the risk of bladder injury. If injury is suspected, infuse the Foley catheter with 250 mL of normal saline to which 50 mg of methylene blue has been added in order to check for a dye leak in the abdomen.

Selected References

Dutta S: Early experience with single incision laparoscopic surgery: eliminating the scar from abdominal operations. *J Pediatr Surg* 44(9):1741-45, 2009.

Horgan S, Cullen JP, Talamini MA, et al: Natural orifice surgery: initial clinical experience. *Surg Endosc* 23(7):1512-18, 2009.

Katsuno G, Nagakari K, Yoshikawa S, et al: Laparoscopic appendectomy for complicated appendicitis: a comparison with open appendectomy. *World J Surg* 33(2):208-14, 2009.

Loh A, Loosemore R, Taylor S, et al: Technique for laparoscopic appendicectomy. *Br J Surg* 79(12):1386-87, 1992.

Smith HF, Fisher RE, Everett ML, et al: Comparative anatomy and phylogenetic distribution of the mammalian cecal appendix. *J Evol Biol* 22(10):1984-99, 2009.

Wei HB, Huang JL, Zheng ZH, et al: Laparoscopic versus open appendectomy: a prospective randomized comparison. *Surg Endosc* 24(2):266-69, 2009.

20

HAND-ASSISTED RIGHT COLECTOMY

Kirk Ludwig and Lauren Kosinski

Step 1. Surgical Anatomy

- ◆ Familiarity with the vascular anatomy of the right colon is essential to the safe conduct of a minimally invasive right colectomy (Figure 20-1). Vascular anatomy also significantly determines resection of colonic malignancies. Several key points guide the laparoscopic surgeon:
  - ▲ Venous and lymphatic drainage run in tandem with named mesenteric arteries.
  - ▲ The ileocolic artery (ICA) branches from the superior mesenteric artery (SMA) just over the duodenum after the take-off of the middle colic artery (MCA). It courses obliquely through the mesocolon to terminate at the cecum, giving off a terminal ileal branch that joins with the small bowel arcade from the SMA.
  - ▲ The right colic artery is usually a branch of the ICA rather than arising from the SMA as is historically depicted.
  - ▲ The MCA proper is typically quite short, branching into two or more arteries (right branch, left branch) just 1 to 2 cm from the aortic origin of the SMA. Rarely is the main MCA itself divided in colon resections. The significant hazard of attempts to control bleeding from a transected main MCA is injury to the SMA.
  - ▲ The branches of the MCA are most easily identified from the cranial aspect of the proximal transverse mesocolon. Once these branches and the adjacent mesocolon are transected, the origin of the ICA can be seen retroperitoneally, as can the more medially oriented SMA.
- ◆ The embryologic fusion plane originates laterally at the white line of Toldt, which occurs where the parietal peritoneum fuses with the visceral peritoneal reflection around the colon and its lateral extension (Figure 20-2). The correct dissection plane is the bloodless embryologic fusion plane. When properly mobilized in this plane, the colon reflects medially on its mesentery to become a nearly midline structure. When the dissection is carried posteriorly past the white line of Toldt, violating the parietal peritoneum as it extends across the retroperitoneal structures, the ureter and gonadal vessels are put at risk and mobilization of the colon is limited.
- ◆ Awareness of the relationships between the cecum, ascending colon, hepatic flexure, and proximal transverse colon to neighboring structures helps to maintain orientation during surgery and prevents injury:

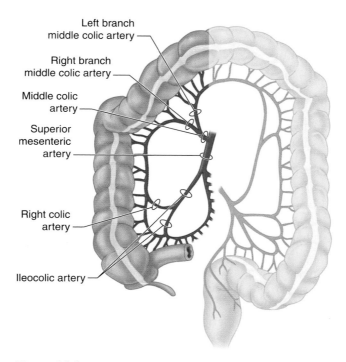

Figure 20-1

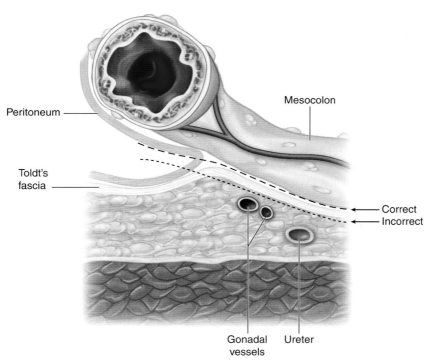

Figure 20-2

▲ The duodenal sweep can be appreciated medial and caudal to the hepatic flexure mesocolon. Risk of injury to the portal triad can be averted by avoiding performance of a Kocher maneuver.

▲ The right kidney and Gerota's fascia are just lateral to the distal ascending colon. Dissection lateral to the embryologic fusion plane can lead to mobilization of the kidney or the second portion of the duodenum (Kocher maneuver).

▲ The right ureter descends retroperitoneally and is not typically exposed unless dissection is carried posterior to the embryologic fusion plane.

▲ The lesser sac must be entered in order to take down the hepatic flexure and transect the transverse mesocolon and MCA branches. The stomach, the gastrocolic, and the hepatocolic ligaments constitute its anterior boundary. Posteriorly, one finds the pancreas and, to the right, the duodenal sweep.

▲ The liver and gallbladder are superior to the hepatocolic ligament. Failure to appreciate this plane can lead to dissection of the porta hepatis.

◆ Surface anatomy considerations principally help with optimal port placement:

▲ Preoperative knowledge of a redundant transverse colon would suggest more caudal placement of the periumbilical hand port incision.

▲ A shift of the hand port site superiorly helps in patients with a relatively long distance between the xiphoid and the umbilicus.

Step 2. Preoperative Considerations

Patient Preparation

◆ Given that the majority of right colectomies are performed for neoplastic diseases (cancer or endoscopically unresectable polyps), staging must be complete before going to the operating room:

▲ A computed tomography (CT) scan of the chest, abdomen, and pelvis is central to the metastatic workup. A positron emission tomography (PET) scan is sometimes also necessary.

▲ The CT scan may also reveal invasion into an adjacent structure, which could preclude a laparoscopic approach.

◆ Lesions must be appropriately localized preoperatively. Although all of the patient's physicians are concerned about making the correct diagnosis, only the surgeon has to perform a resection and must manage the technical details of this procedure:

▲ Review the colonoscopy report; note the expected location of the target lesion and the presence and character (including pathology report) of any other lesions.

▲ Tattoos are critical for smaller or nonpalpable lesions. Note the type of dye used (India ink lasts, methylene blue disperses).

▲ Review of imaging studies (CT, barium enema) may help with localization.

- ▲ Colonoscopy must be repeated if the following occurs:
  - Tumor location is unclear from the report.
  - There is a discrepancy between imaging studies and colonoscopy reports.
  - There are additional lesions that may require resection.
- ◆ Plan the extent of resection with regard to both margins and vascular ligation:
  - ▲ The right branch of the MCA should be included for resection of neoplasms of the cecum or the proximal ascending colon.
  - ▲ For neoplasms of the hepatic flexure or proximal transverse colon, all the MCA branches (or the trunk) must be included.
  - ▲ For inflammatory bowel disease or other benign indications, there is no need to perform a high ligation of the arteries or regional lymphadenectomy.
- ◆ Past surgical history and an abdominal examination may reveal risks that could present challenges to a minimally invasive approach:
  - ▲ Surgical scars and history of adhesions or bowel obstruction may alter port site placement or technique of entry.
  - ▲ The presence of a ventral hernia or abdominal wall mesh could also change the approach.
  - ▲ The size of a tumor or inflammatory mass could preclude extraction through a hand port.
  - ▲ Several studies have suggested that preoperative bowel preparation is not necessary for elective colon resection. However, the difficulty of manipulating a stool-laden colon laparoscopically and the problems controlling spillage should the colon be violated during resection lead us to recommend formal bowel preparation.
- ◆ Formal stoma marking should be made preoperatively if there is a chance that an ileostomy will be created.

Equipment and Instrumentation

- ◆ Use of a 5-mm scope and instruments affords the most flexibility.
- ◆ A 30-degree scope is best, although it does take more skill and experience to use well.

Anesthesia

- Prophylactic antibiotics are given to cover gram-negative and anaerobic organisms preoperatively. Coverage is extended postoperatively only for special situations.
- Prophylactic anticoagulation is used unless there are specific contraindications.
- An orogastric tube is placed by anesthesia to decompress the stomach.

Room Setup and Patient Positioning

- The room setup is depicted in Figure 20-3:
  - ▲ Attend to the position of the operating table and room setup before the case begins.
  - ▲ Place monitors first, because laparoscopic surgery is image-oriented surgery.
  - ▲ Place the instrument tower next and lights last.
- There are a few key features of patient positioning:
  - ▲ The patient is supine.
  - ▲ Both arms will be tucked in a draw sheet on which the patient lies to help secure the patient to the table; the anesthesiologist may need to adjust oxygen saturation monitoring and IV placement accordingly. Three-inch silk tape or Velcro strips are placed across the chest and lower extremities to help stabilize the patient even when the table is tilted strongly to assist with operative exposure.
  - ▲ Sequential compression devices are placed.
  - ▲ The patient's abdomen is prepared and draped widely. An Ioban sheet is positioned to hold towels in place.
  - ▲ All cords are run off the operating room table together to the tower in a bundle. This simplifies the work area and enables easier movement around the table.

Step 3. Operative Steps

- Access and port placement:
  - ▲ The hand port template is used to demarcate the incision length, which should be no larger than the surgeon's glove size (e.g., size 7 glove would require a 6- to 7-cm hand port incision).
  - ▲ The hand port incision is centered on the point that is half way between the anterior superior iliac crest and the costal margin. The incision may be quite a bit above the umbilicus in an obese patient.
  - ▲ The hand port incision is made first, and the hand-assist device is placed.
  - ▲ A 12-mm port is advanced through the hand port for insufflation (15 mmHg).
  - ▲ Two additional ports (5 mm each) are placed. The subxiphoid port is placed just to the left of the midline (farther left if an extended right hemicolectomy is anticipated). The left upper quadrant port is placed at the midclavicular line, halving the distance between the costal margin and the superior end of the hand port incision (Figure 20-4).

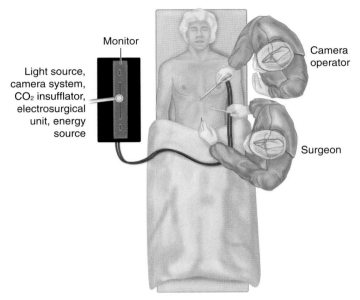

Monitor

Light source,
camera system,
CO$_2$ insufflator,
electrosurgical
unit, energy
source

Camera
operator

Surgeon

Figure 20-3

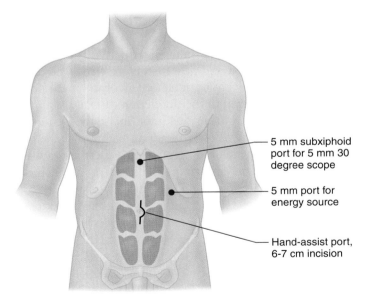

5 mm subxiphoid
port for 5 mm 30
degree scope

5 mm port for
energy source

Hand-assist port,
6-7 cm incision

Figure 20-4

- ◆ Abdominal survey:
  - ▲ Mobilize the falciform ligament if it interferes with the subxiphoid port.
  - ▲ Evaluate the liver and peritoneum for metastases in a cancer resection.
  - ▲ Identify the target lesion.
- ◆ Mobilization of the colon:
  - ▲ This is a top down approach. The anatomy is viewed from above and the dissection moves from the right upper quadrant to the right lower quadrant. Mobilization of the anatomy involves lifting the bowel and its mesentery up off of the retroperitoneum.
  - ▲ Mobilization of the colon begins in the lesser sac. First, we divide the gastrocolic and hepatocolic ligaments to enter the lesser sac and expose the ventral surface of the transverse mesocolon.
  - ▲ The duodenal sweep and hepatic flexure will come into view laterally.
  - ▲ As the dissection is carried to the patient's right, Gerota's fascia also comes into view.
  - ▲ Leave the lateral attachments in place initially and expose the rest of the duodenum first by dividing filmy attachments between the ascending mesocolon and duodenum.
  - ▲ Divide the lateral attachments of the right colon, carrying the dissection medially along the embryologic fusion plane. Failure to dissect in this avascular plane will result in exposure of the right psoas muscle, ureter, and gonadal vessels. Alternatively, the right kidney may be mobilized or a Kocher maneuver may inadvertently be performed.
  - ▲ Eventually, the entire right colon and ileal mesentery will be elevated off of the retroperitoneum, leaving only the embryologic attachments of the small bowel mesentery attached from the right lower quadrant up to the duodenum. Finally, with the ileal mesentery and small bowel draped into the left lower quadrant, incise the peritoneum at the base of the ileal mesentery from the right lower quadrant back up to the duodenum/ligament of Trietz. This will later allow the ileum to easily come up into the wound for exteriorization and anastomosis. specimen and performing the extracorporeal anastomosis.
- ◆ The lymphovascular pedicles are identified and divided (Figure 20-5):
  - ▲ Find the middle colic vessels near their origin by holding the transverse colon in the palm, elevate it, and use the index finger and thumb to palpate the base of the transverse mesocolon. One or more branches of the MCA will be divided depending on the extent of the resection. A bipolar vessel sealing (device can be used to divide the mesentery and vessels just caudal to the pancreas. Leave a stump of vessel behind in case there is bleeding so that a vascular load of a stapler Endostapler or an Endoloop can be applied.
  - ▲ Identify the ileocolic artery sharply to the left of the line of MCA middle colic artery transection.
  - ▲ Confirm the identity of the ICA iliocolic artery:

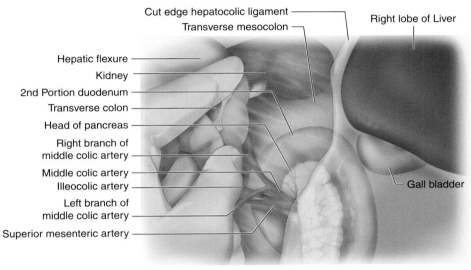

Cut edge hepatocolic ligament

Transverse mesocolon

Right lobe of Liver

Hepatic flexure

Kidney

2nd Portion duodenum

Transverse colon

Head of pancreas

Right branch of
middle colic artery

Middle colic artery

Illeocolic artery

Left branch of
middle colic artery

Superior mesenteric artery

Gall bladder

Figure 20-5

- Retract the transverse colon superiorly and return the hepatic flexure to its natural position in the right upper quadrant.
- Tent the ICA by retracting the cecum caudally and to the patient's right.
- Divide the ICA near its origin leaving a 2-cm pedicle; do this from the superior vantage point (retract transverse colon inferiorly again).
- About 90% of the time the right colic artery is a branch of the ICA.
  - ▲ If the vessels are highly calcified, use a vascular load of the laparoscopic stapler.
  - ▲ Divide the mesentery from the junction of the ICA and SMA to the marginal artery along the ileum.
- Desufflate the abdomen through the ports. This is particularly important in cancer resections to avoid seeding port sites with aerosolized tumor cells.
- Exteriorize the right colon through the gel port:
  - ▲ Divide the ileum and the transverse colon externally using a handheld linear cutting stapler.
- Perform an ileocolic anastomosis. This can be done as for conventional open resections. Take care to avoid twisting the ileum, especially if it was divided intracorporally. Return bowel to the abdomen.
- *Examine the specimen to be sure the target lesion is in the specimen.*
- Close the incisions. No fascial closure is required for the 5-mm ports. Close the skin with a 4-0 absorbable deep dermal running suture followed by application of a wound sealant.

Step 4. Postoperative Care

- A fast-track plan is encouraged.
- *Analgesia.* A PCA pump or Toradol with intermittent parenteral narcotics can be used, transitioning promptly to oral analgesics once solid food is started.
- *Nasogastric tube.* This is not routinely used unless there is extensive lysis of adhesions.
- *Diet.* Clear liquids are offered on postoperative day 1 and a soft diet on postoperative day 2 unless the patient has nausea, vomiting, distention, or significant belching.
- *Urinary catheter.* This is removed on postoperative day 1 or 2.
- *Activity.* The patient is encouraged to sit or stand at the bedside the day of surgery and to sit in a chair the morning following surgery. Ambulation is ordered on postoperative day 1.
- *Discharge.* The patient can be discharged once a diet is tolerated and bowel function has resumed. This usually happens by postoperative day 3 to 5.

Step 5. Pearls and Pitfalls

- The learning curve for laparoscopic colon resection can be shortened by utilizing the hand-assisted approach:
  - ▲ It is estimated that one must perform 25 to 50 pure laparoscopic colon resections to become proficient.
  - ▲ Hand-assisted laparoscopic surgery (HALS) allows the surgeon to work with less experienced staff. Bowel retraction and vessel identification and division (especially of the middle colic artery) are easier.
- The goal of the operation is to perform a safe operation (and a curative operation in the setting of cancer). Patients need a *good* operation, not necessarily a laparoscopic one.
- A periumbilical hand port incision is preferred to a Pfannenstiel incision for several reasons.
- Mobilization of the mesocolon around the duodenum should involve gentle, posterior displacement of the duodenum. Care should be taken to avoid mobilization of the duodenum (the Kocher maneuver) to avoid exposure of the porta hepatis and risk of injury to those structures.
- Avoid the temptation to ligate the vascular pedicles extracorporally. It's never possible to reach the mesentery well once bowel is exteriorized, and it's harder to control bleeding.
- Taking at least one branch of the middle colic artery helps assure good length of exteriorized transverse colon and avoid traction injury of the middle colic artery when exteriorizing the bowel.
- Leave a short stump of vessel behind when dividing vessels with a vessel sealing and cutting device.
- Adhesions in the lesser sac (fusion of the gastrocolic or hepatocolic ligaments with the retroperitoneum or adhesions between the posterior stomach and retroperitoneum) can interfere with adequate exposure of the transverse mesocolon and safe identification of the middle colic artery.
- Hand-assisted laparoscopic surgery is still image-based surgery. The hand is a sophisticated retraction device.
- This procedure safely handles bowel and protects it from the power source.
- Manipulation can thin tissue and help identify vessels.
- Typically, the index finger leads the way, the next three fingers provide retraction, and the thumb provides countertraction.

Selected References

Cima RR, Pattana-arun J, Larson DW, et al: Experience with 969 minimal access colectomies: the role of hand-assisted laparoscopy in expanding minimally invasive surgery for complex colectomies. *J Am Coll Surg* 206(5):946-50, 2008; discussion 950-52.

Hassan I, You YN, Cima RR, et al: Hand-assisted versus laparoscopic-assisted colorectal surgery: practice patterns and clinical outcomes in a minimally-invasive colorectal practice. *Surg Endosc* 22(3):739-43, 2008.

Lee SW, Yoo J, Dujovny N, et al: Laparoscopic vs. hand-assisted laparoscopic sigmoidectomy for diverticulitis. *Dis Colon Rectum* 49(4): 464-69, 2006.

Marcello PW, Fleshman JW, Milsom JW, et al: Hand-assisted laparoscopic vs. laparoscopic colorectal surgery: a multicenter, prospective, randomized trial. *Dis Colon Rectum* 51(6):818-26, 2008; discussion 826-28.

Ringley C, Lee YK, Iqbal A, et al: Comparison of conventional laparoscopic and hand-assisted oncologic segmental colonic resection. *Surg Endosc* 21(12):2137-41, 2007.

Stein S, Whelan RL. The controversy regarding hand-assisted colorectal resection. *Surg Endosc* 21(12):2123-26, 2007.

Targarona EM, Gracia E, Garriga J, et al: Prospective randomized trial comparing conventional laparoscopic colectomy with hand-assisted laparoscopic colectomy: applicability, immediate clinical outcome, inflammatory response, and cost. *Surg Endosc* 16(2):234-39, 2002.

Yamaguchi S, Kuroyanagi H, Milsom JW, et al: Venous anatomy of the right colon: precise structure of the major veins and gastrocolic trunk in 58 cadavers. *Dis Colon Rectum* 45(10):1337-40, 2002.

21

RIGHT HEMICOLECTOMY

Jennifer L. Irani and David C. Brooks

Step 1. Surgical Anatomy

- The ileocolic vascular pedicle of the superior mesenteric artery must be isolated and divided. If the resection is performed for malignancy, it is important to divide this pedicle close to the root of the mesentery.
- The mesenteric vessels should be divided up to and including the right branch of the middle colic artery for a formal right hemicolectomy.
- The duodenum must be identified and protected.

Step 2. Preoperative Considerations

Patient Preparation

- A preoperative colonoscopy will identify the lesion to be removed. The endoscopist should tattoo the lesion in order to allow the operating surgeon to then identify a mucosal lesion from the serosal side of the bowel, and thus remove the appropriate specimen.
- An abdominal computed tomography (CT) scan may also help localize the lesion to be removed as well as provide an anatomic overview of the patient's abdomen.
- A full preoperative metastatic workup should be performed for malignant lesions.
- Patients should receive preoperative bowel preparation the day before surgery (e.g., GoLYTELY, HalfLytely, phospho soda, magnesium citrate).
- Within 1 hour of skin incision, intravenous (IV) antibiotics must be administered.
- Indications for laparoscopic right colectomy are the same as those for open colectomy and include colonic polyps, Crohn disease, colon cancer, and so on.
- Oncologic results have been shown to be equivalent between laparoscopic and open surgery for colon cancer.
- There are some contraindications to laparoscopic colectomy, which include the following:
  - ▲ T4 disease (tumor extension into an adjacent organ)

▲ Resectable metastatic disease requiring resection of adjacent organs
▲ Bowel perforation or obstruction or fistula (e.g., Crohn disease)
▲ Coagulopathy
▲ Multiple prior abdominal surgeries/adhesions (relative contraindication)

Equipment and Instrumentation

Laparoscopic right hemicolectomy is carried out using standard laparoscopic instruments, including atraumatic bowel graspers and scissors with electrocautery attachment:

• Veress needle, 12-mm port, 5-mm ports.
• A 5-mm or 10-mm, 30-degree camera (a zero-degree camera can also be used).
• Wound protector.
• 5-mm LigaSure device (Covidien, Mansfield, Massachusetts) or Harmonic scalpel (Ethicon, Somerville, New Jersey).
• Endo GIA (Autosuture, Covidien) roticulating stapler with gastrointestinal (3.5-mm staple height) cartridge load for division of colon; a cartridge (2.5-mm staple height) for division of ileum and a vascular cartridge (2-mm staple height) can be used for division of ileocolic vascular pedicle instead of using one of the cutting or sealing devices LigaSure or Harmonic scalpel.
• An Endoloop (Ethicon, Somerville, New Jersey) should be available (although not necessarily opened) in case of the need for rapid vascular control.
• Laparoscopic suction/irrigator.
• Handheld linear cutting gastrointestinal stapler (3.5-mm staple height).
• Handheld linear non-cutting TA gastrointestinal stapler (3.5- to 4.8-mm staple height).

Anesthesia

- Given the limited incisions, preoperative epidural placement is rarely required:
  - ▲ General anesthesia is administered, and the patient is intubated with a regular endotracheal tube.
  - ▲ A nasogastric tube is placed for gastric decompression.
  - ▲ A Foley catheter is placed.
- Venodynes or subcutaneous heparin is administered for deep venous thrombosis (DVT) prophylaxis.
- Preoperative antibiotics are administered prior to skin incision.

Room Setup and Patient Positioning

- The patient is positioned supine with both arms tucked at the side (at a minimum, left arm must be tucked), ensuring adequate padding of pressure points. A safety strap is put in place.

Step 3. Operative Steps

Access and Port Placement

- A Veress needle is inserted in the left upper quadrant and pneumoperitoneum is established with carbon dioxide to a pressure of approximately 15 mmHg.
- A 12-mm port is inserted in the supraumbilical region, and a 30-degree camera is introduced.
- The abdomen is inspected for metastatic disease, especially focusing on the liver.
- Insert a 5-mm port in the left lower quadrant, left upper quadrant, and subxiphoid region under direct vision (Figure 21-1).

Dissection

- Adhesions, if present, are gently taken down using sharp dissection, and the abdomen is further explored for metastasis and resectability.
- The patient is positioned in Trendelenburg with the left side down.
- Dissection begins by identifying the appendix, cecum, and terminal ileum. The assistant provides medial traction of the cecum.
- The right colon lateral attachments are then taken down. Identify and sharply incise the right white line of Toldt, beginning at the cecum, taking care to identify and avoid the right ureter (Figure 21-2).
- The sharp dissection continues up to and around the hepatic flexure while the assistant is providing medial traction on the right colon. The patient is placed in reverse Trendelenburg to facilitate exposure. The duodenum is protected at all times. When the right colon is retracted medially, the duodenum is identified (Figure 21-3).

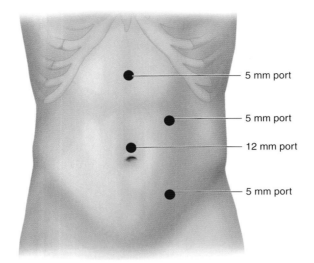

5 mm port

5 mm port

12 mm port

5 mm port

Figure 21-1

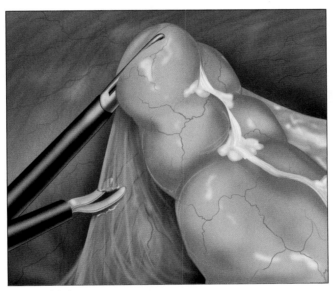

Figure 21-2

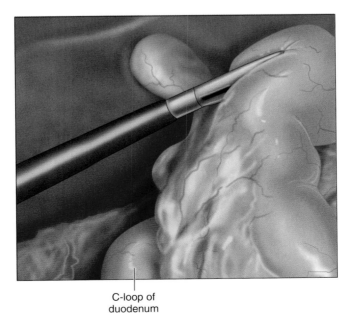

C-loop of
duodenum

Figure 21-3

Division of Bowel and Vascular Pedicle

◆ Once the right colon is medialized, divide the terminal ileum using a laparoscopic stapler (Figure 21-4A).
◆ It is best to divide the mesentery using a LigaSure or ultrasonic coagulator to maintain hemostasis while minimizing thermal spread. The ileocolic and right colic vessels may be divided with these devices. Ensure proximal ligation of vessels for malignant disease to encompass the maximum number of lymph nodes in the specimen (Figure 21-5).
◆ Isolate and clear the distal resection line on the transverse colon. Divide the colon with a laparoscopic stapler (Figure 21-4B).

Specimen Removal

◆ The specimen is placed in the right upper quadrant, and the patient is placed in the neutral position.
◆ Either the subxiphoid or the umbilical port site is used for specimen extraction and extracorporeal anastomosis.
◆ The port is removed and the site is extended for 4 cm vertically. A wound protector may be used at this point. When the specimen is removed, the proximal and distal segments of bowel are brought out through the wound.

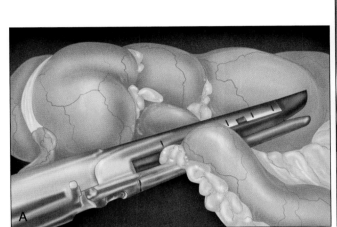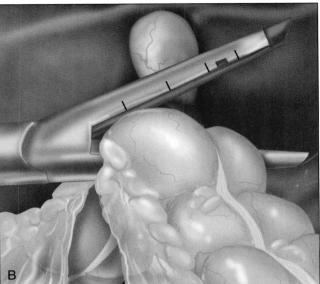

Figure 21-4 A, B

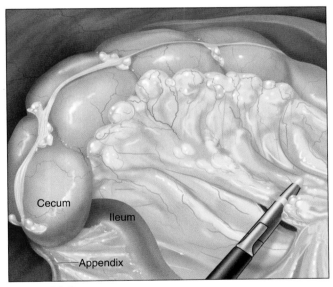

Figure 21-5

Anastomosis

- A side-to-side, functional end-to-end anastomosis is performed with a handheld linear stapler GIA stapler, and the common enterotomy is closed with a TA stapler. The anastomosis is returned to the abdomen.
- The 4-cm incision is closed. Pneumoperitoneum is reestablished, and the abdomen is inspected for bleeding.
- All ports are removed under direct vision, irrigated, and closed.

Step 4. Postoperative Care

- Postoperative care following laparoscopic right colectomy is the same as that for open colectomy. Await return of bowel function, adequate PO intake, and pain control prior to discharge.

Step 5. Pearls and Pitfalls

- Move the camera and instruments around to achieve triangulation.
- Always know the location of the right ureter, duodenum, IVC, and stomach to avoid inadvertent injury.
- Upsize ports if necessary to accommodate cameras and staplers as needed.
- Closely visualize the abdomen for bleeding as pneumoperitoneum is being released.

Selected References

The Clinical Outcomes of Surgical Therapy Study Group: A comparison of laparoscopically assisted and open colectomy for colon cancer. *N Engl J Med* 350(20):2050-59, 2004.
Davies MM, Nelson H: Small bowel/colon resection. In Zinner MJ, Ashley SW (editors): Maingot's Abdominal Operations, 11th ed. New York, McGraw-Hill, 2007, pp. 1151-1167.
Larson DW, Nelson H: Laparoscopic colectomy for cancer. *J Gastrointest Surg* 8(5):636-42, 2004.

CHAPTER 22

LEFT COLON RESECTION (MEDIAL TO LATERAL APPROACH)

Mark H. Whiteford

Step 1. Surgical Anatomy

- The left colon receives arterial input via the inferior mesenteric artery (IMA). Soon after its takeoff from the abdominal aorta, the IMA branches into a left (descending) colic branch and the superior hemorrhoidal artery (SHA). The SHA continues down to the rectum, along the way giving off sigmoidal branches.
- The venous drainage of the left colon is into the inferior mesenteric vein (IMV), which passes posterolateral to the IMA, parallel to the aorta in a cephalad direction, to pass under the tail of the pancreas where it joins the splenic vein.
- The lymphatic drainage follows the arteries.
- The sympathetic plexus interdigitates around the aorta at the base of the IMA, then it coalesces into the left and right hypogastric nerves as they course over the common iliacs and into the pelvis.
- The left ureter and gonadal vessels lie in the retroperitoneum posterior to the left colon mesentery.

Step 2. Preoperative Considerations

Patient Preparation

- The most common indications for laparoscopic left colectomy are cancer, polyps, and diverticulitis.

Equipment and Instrumentation

- Laparoscopic instrumentation includes scissors, atraumatic graspers, Maryland dissector, suction cautery, vessel-sealing device, laparoscopic and open stapling devices.
- Open instrumentation should be available for fashioning the anastomosis and in the event of conversion.

Anesthesia

- Indications for bowel preparation, perioperative antibiotics, and deep venous prophylaxis are the same for laparoscopic as for open approaches.
- Urinary catheter is inserted.

Room Setup and Patient Positioning

- Following induction of general endotracheal anesthesia, the patient is placed in a neutral lithotomy position on a well-padded electric operating room table.
- Shoulders, hips and knees should be in the same plane. Arms are carefully padded and tucked at the sides using an oversized beanbag or tucked with sheets. Chest straps or tapes may be placed for added security.
- The surgeon and camera operator stand on the patient's right, assistant on the left (Figure 22-1).

Step 3. Operative Steps

Access and Port Placement

- Following port placement, laparoscopic exploration and any necessary adhesiolysis, the patient is placed in a steep Trendelenburg position with the right side tilted down.

Establish plane between the superior hemorrhoidal artery and the sacral promontory:
- The small bowel is swept up out of the pelvis and off to the right upper quadrant. The base of the medial (right side of the sigmoid) mesentery over the sacral promontory is exposed by placing the sigmoid mesocolon on anterolateral traction toward the left. The peritoneum over the root of the sigmoid mesentery is scored parallel to and just posterior to the arc of the superior hemorrhoidal artery as it courses over the sacral promontory. This is extended from the sacral hollow up to the root of the IMA (Figure 22-2).

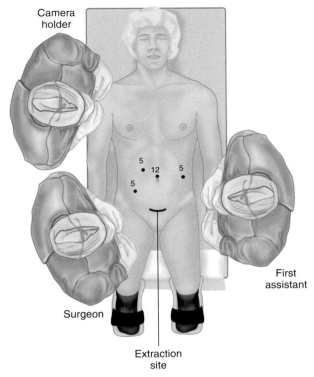

Camera holder

Surgeon

First assistant

Extraction site

Figure 22-1

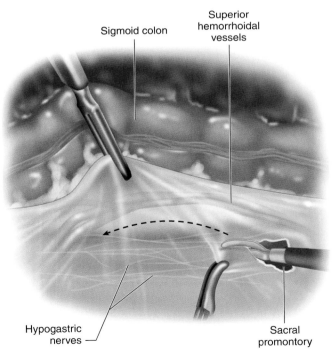

Sigmoid colon

Superior hemorrhoidal vessels

Hypogastric nerves

Sacral promontory

Figure 22-2

- With a gentle blunt anterior to posterior sweeping motion, the areolar, avascular retroperi- toneal plane is created. The hypogastric nerves are identified and preserved posteriorly.
- Once established, the purplish areolar plane between the sigmoid colon mesentery and the retroperitoneal structures is swept down. This creates a "cave," which will be deepened up and out to the lateral abdominal sidewall. The left ureter should be identified just lateral to the aorta then coursing down over the left iliac vessels. If it is not visible, the dissection plane may have been too posterior, resulting in the ureter inadvertently being swept anteriorly with the mesosigmoid. If so, the ureter must be identified, freed, then swept posteriorly (Figure 22-3).

Identification and ligation of the inferior mesenteric artery and vein:
- With the retroperitoneal plane established, the ureter and gonadal vessels preserved, and the dissection complete out to the white line of Toldt, the next step is to continue the plane cranially and medially to identify the inferior mesenteric artery (IMA).
- The inferior mesenteric vein (IMV) runs posterolateral then cephalad to the IMA, continuing parallel to the aorta before passing behind the ligament of Treitz and the tail of the pancreas.
- An avascular window exists between the IMV and aorta between the IMA and the ligament of Treitz (Figure 22-4).
- For colorectal cancer, where a high vascular ligation is preferred, this window can be entered to isolate and divide the root of the IMA.

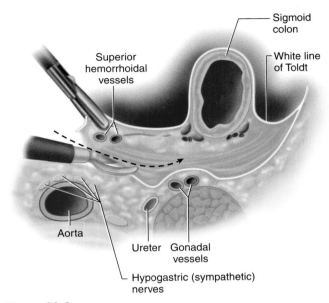

Figure 22-3

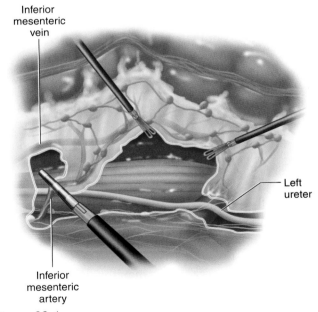

Figure 22-4

- For diverticular disease, vascular ligation may be performed distal to the left colic artery. Our preference for vascular control is to utilize a laparoscopic 5-mm vessel-sealing device (Figure 22-5).
- The IMV is then isolated and divided in a similar fashion. The descending colon mesentery can now be elevated and dissected off of Gerota's fascia out to the lateral attachments and up behind the splenic flexure. The cephalad extent of retroperitoneal dissection is to the inferior edge of the pancreas.

Division of the lateral attachments and splenic flexure:
- The sigmoid colon is retracted medially and the white line of Toldt divided starting at the sigmoid colon and progressing proximally.
- Splenic flexure mobilization can be facilitated by repositioning the patient in reverse Trendelenburg and by using a vessel-sealing device to maintain hemostasis. The plane of dissection is maintained between the colonic wall and the greater omentum. The proximal extent of the dissection should be into the lesser sac up to the level of the midtransverse colon (Figure 22-6).
- Omental attachments to the superior aspect of the splenic flexure mesentery are likewise released. This should provide an adequate length of colon for most pelvic anastomoses.

Division of the mesorectum and rectum:
- The patient is repositioned back into steep Trendelenburg and attention directed back into the pelvis. Distal dissection is continued posterior to the rectum along the previously established planes between the fascia propria of the mesorectum and the presacral fascia (Figure 22-7).
- Left lateral peritoneal attachments of the rectosigmoid colon are released down to the distal resection margin.
- The mesorectum is divided using a vessel-sealing device (Figure 22-8).
- The rectum is divided using an endoscopic stapler.
- Alternatively, these last steps can be performed with open techniques via an extraction incision in the lower abdomen.

Specimen exteriorization, resection, and colorectal anastomosis:
- A 6- to 8-cm Pfannenstiel or lower midline extraction incision is created and a wound protector placed.
- The left colon is delivered. Its mesentery is divided just proximal to the IMA transection site. The bowel is divided. An end-to-end anastomosis (EEA) anvil is secured in the end of healthy descending colon. The fashioning of a transanal EEA anastomosis is monitored directly through the extraction site or alternatively the extraction site is closed, pneumoperitoneum reestablished, and the anastomosis monitored through laparoscopic techniques.
- An anastomotic air leak test is performed, followed by an inspection of the dissection planes for hemostasis.
- Trocars and extraction sites are closed using absorbable sutures.

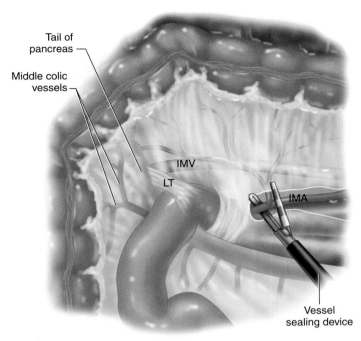

Figure 22-5

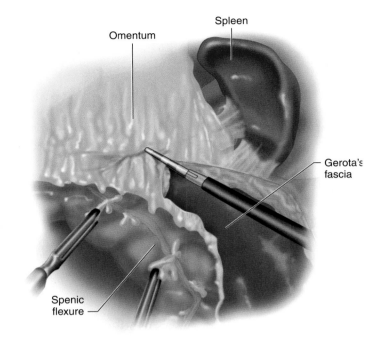

Figure 22-6

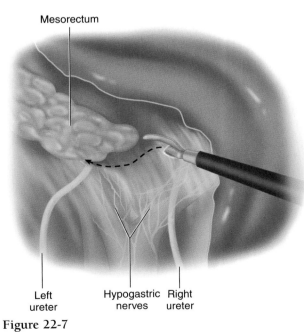

Figure 22-7

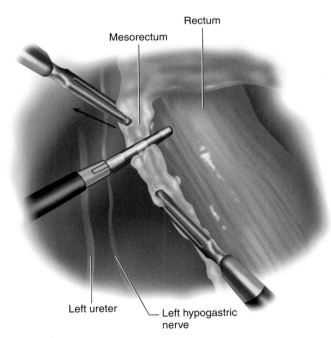

Figure 22-8

Step 4. Postoperative Care

- Laparoscopic colorectal surgery is particularly suited for enhanced recovery programs.
- We encourage early postoperative feeding and ambulation.
- Nasogastric tubes and surgical drains are not used and urinary catheters are removed on postoperative day 1.

Step 5. Pearls and Pitfalls

- Recent research has called into question the need for routine cathartic bowel preparation for elective colon surgery. Our practice has likewise moved away from routine bowel preparation with some exceptions. These include when intraoperative colonoscopy for tumor localization, anastomosis with covering ostomy, and total mesorectal excision are planned, or when the patient has such a heavy fecal load that it will overwhelm the delicate laparoscopic instruments (i.e., total colectomy for chronic constipation).
- Laparoscopic surgery does not afford the surgeon the ability to use his or her hand to palpate and locate small polyps or tumors. Therefore, when operating for these indications, preoperative colonoscopy with three-quadrant submucosal injection of tattooing substance just distal to the lesion is the preferred technique. The availability of intraoperative colonoscopy is also ideal when the patient is bowel prepped and the lesion cannot be identified using laparoscopic techniques.
- The splenic flexure mobilization is usually approached in a retrograde fashion as described earlier. A compliment to this approach is to mobilize laterally just up to the flexure then move to the midtransverse colon. The omentum can be elevated cephalad and a plane between the omentum and transverse colon created up into the lesser sac. Once the lesser sac is opened, this plane is continued distally along the colon and mesocolon to complete the splenic flexure mobilization.

Selected References

Milsom JW, Böhm B, Nakajima K: *Laparoscopic Colorectal Surgery,* 2nd ed. New York, Springer, 2006.

23

Total Proctocolectomy with Ileal-Pouch Anal Anastomosis

Robert R. Cima, David W. Larson, and Eric J. Dozois

Step 1. Surgical Anatomy

- Chronic ulcerative colitis (CUC) is an inflammatory bowel disease limited to the mucosa of the rectum and colon. Although no etiologic factor has been identified, population studies suggest there is both a genetic and an environmental component contributing to the development of CUC. The disease course is characterized by intermittent flares of disease activity. Medical therapy for the intestinal manifestations of CUC is directed at controlling symptoms by modulating the inflammatory process. To date, no medical therapy is curative. However, surgical removal of the colon and rectum cures the intestinal manifestations of the disease and eliminates or markedly reduces the associated risk of malignancy in long-standing CUC. Surgical intervention for CUC is divided into two broad categories, emergent and elective, that will influence the type of surgery performed. Emergency operations are directed at life-threatening complications of CUC and are not intended as definitive surgical treatment for CUC. Alternatively, elective surgery is intended as a definitive treatment for the intestinal symptoms. In appropriately selected patients, the best surgical option is the total proctocolectomy with an ileal pouch-anal anastomosis (IPAA). The IPAA avoids the need for a permanent stoma while maintaining the normal route of defecation.
- This is a technically demanding operation and should be performed by surgeons comfortable with both the technical aspects of the procedure and management of the many possible complications. Traditionally, this complex operation has been performed through a midline laparotomy. However, improved technology and increased surgical experience with advanced laparoscopy have permitted a number of surgeons and centers to offer a minimally invasive approach to the IPAA procedure. Although the initial laparoscopic IPAA experience was characterized by long operative times, experience and new technology have significantly reduced operative times while maintaining the safety and clinical outcomes, making the laparoscopic IPAA comparable to the open procedure.

Step 2. Preoperative Considerations

Patient Preparation

- In chronic ulcerative colitis (CUC) patients with fulminant or toxic disease, the appropriate choice of operation is a total abdominal colectomy with Hartmann pouch and end ileostomy. This operation removes the majority of the diseased organ, allows the patient to be tapered off of all immunosuppressive medications, and regain their health and nutritional status before proceeding to a definitive restorative operation (IPAA).
- Prior to proceeding to an IPAA, the diagnosis of CUC or indeterminate colitis needs to be firmly established. Crohn's disease is a considered a significant contraindication for proceeding to an IPAA.
- Patients need to visit with an enterostomal therapist for pre-operative stoma marking and to begin education regarding the care of the stoma. Using a laparoscopic approach for an IPAA results in a significantly shortened length of stay in hospital and decreases the opportunity for education regarding stoma management.
- We do not routinely use oral antibiotics nor a mechanical bowel preparation as it tends to cause bowel distension with liquid stool which makes colon manipulation more difficult. Each patient receives one or two tap water enemas the morning of operation.
- The operating room requirements for an efficient laparoscopic TPC-IPAA include:
  - ▲ an electronically controlled operating table with a significant range in side to side tilt and steep Trendlenberg and reverse Trendlenberg capability to facilitate the use of gravity to move the small intestine out of the way of dissection.
  - ▲ a non-skid operating table surface to minimize patient movement on the table during the numerous position changes. This reduces the risk of the patient sliding off of the table as well as shear injury to the patient's skin which can predispose to pressure related skin breakdown. An alternative approach is to use a "bean bag."
  - ▲ a minimum of three video monitors, preferably four, are available for use during the case with two positioned off the shoulders of the patient and one at the foot of the table.
  - ▲ ideally all the equipment should be off the floor attached to ceiling booms which permit easier movement of equipment during the procedure.
- All patients require a padded chest strap placed securing them to the table. They need to be positioned in modified Lloyd-Davies lithotomy with both arms padded, protected, and tucked against their torso. The patient's legs are placed in leg holder that allows the hips and thighs to be flat with respect to the abdomen but the lower leg to be positioned downward (i.e. Yellofin® Stirrups, Allen® Medical Systems). These leg holders minimize the chance of patient movement on the table during positioning changes as well as permitting access to the perineum for placement of a circular stapler or a vaginal retractor/manipulator.
- In patients who have recently received or are currently on steroids, a brief pulse of steroids is appropriate during the peri-operative period.

Anesthesia

- Prior to incision, sequential compression devices are placed on the calves, an orogastric tube and urinary catheter are placed and intravenous antibiotics and H2 blockers and subcutaneous heparin are administered.

Room Setup and Patient Positioning

- The patient is placed in the modified lithotomy with both arms padded, protected, and tucked against the torso. It is important that the thighs are positioned in such a way that they are level with the abdomen. A chest strap is applied to minimize the risk of the patient shifting on the operating table during frequent position changes during the procedure. Ideally, video monitors are available on movable booms to permit placement above the patient's left and right shoulders and one in the area between the patient's legs during different phases of the operation.

Step 3. Operative Steps

Laparoscopically-Assisted (LA) Approach

- A diamond configuration for trocar placement is used. Four trocars, three 5-mm and one 10–12-mm are placed.
- A 10-12 mm trocar is placed in the future ileostomy site after an open technique is used to enter the abdomen. Pneumoperitoneum is established and laparoscopic exploration of the abdomen is undertaken with a 5 mm 30 degree laparoscope to assess the feasibility of proceeding with a minimally invasive approach.
- Extensive adhesions, unanticipated anatomic or inflammatory processes that preclude a minimally invasive should prompt immediate conversion to an open procedure.
- The remaining 5-mm trocars are placed under direct vision in a diamond configuration with one in the left lower quadrant, one in the midline in the suprapubic position, and the last one in the midline above the umbilicus (Fig. 23-1).
- During the procedure, the first assistant is always standing across from the surgeon while the camera operator is positioned next to the surgeon. For the majority of the procedure, the camera will be used in supraumbilical trocar.

Left Colon Mobilization

- The patient is placed in maximal Trendelenburg with the left side elevated 30-degrees. The surgeon is positioned on the patient's right side with the camera operator standing next to the surgeon closest to the patient's head. The camera is placed in the midline supra-umbilical trocar.
- The surgeon will be using the right lower and suprapubic trocars to begin the mobilization of the left colon. The white line of Toldt is incised, reflecting the left colon medially as it is freed from the lateral peritoneal attachments (Figure 23-6). The laparoscopic retractor is used from the right lower quadrant trocar while the dissector is in the suprapubic position.
- A critical step during this portion of the operation is identification of the left ureter. It is important to mobilize the colon in the appropriate plane which close to the colonic border as it is quite easy to dissect behind the kidney.
- The mobilization of the sigmoid and left colon is considered complete when it is medial to left ureter along its entire course.
- The distal aspect of the splenic flexure can be mobilized while the patient is in this position. However, to complete the mobilization the patient is repositioned into reverse Trendelenburg while maintaining the left side elevated.
- To facilitate dissecting more proximally on the transverse colon, the surgeon moves between the patient's leg to utilize the suprapubic and left lower quadrant trocars. The camera operator remains on the patient's right side while the assistant moves to the right side to use the right lower quadrant trocar site to provide retraction of the omentum upward while the surgeon retracts down into the abdomen.
- The splenic flexure is mobilized off Gerota's fascia and the tail of the pancreas. Once the flexure has been fully mobilized from the lateral aspect, the lesser sac must be completely opened. (Fig 23-3) This ensures that distal transverse colon and splenic flexure can be brought to the umbilicus to facilitate extraction of the specimen if extra-corporeal vessel division is utilized.

Right Colon Mobilization

- Once the left colon and splenic flexure are mobilized, attention is turned to the mobilizing the right colon, hepatic flexure, and the small bowel mesentery.
- The patient is once again placed in maximal Trendelenburg with the right side elevated approximately 30 degrees.
- The surgeon and camera operator move to the patient's left side. The small bowel is retracted into the left upper quadrant.
- Using a grasper through the left lower quadrant trocar the terminal ileum and cecum are retracted up and toward the left upper abdomen.
- The dissecting instrument is placed through the suprapubic trocar. The peritoneum surrounding the terminal ileum and cecum is incised to reveal the retroperitoneal plane and underlying structures.
- Similar to the left side it is extremely important to identify and protect the right ureter.
- The right colon is dissected free from the lateral peritoneal attachments. Once the lateral attachments are divided attention is turned to completing the mobilization of the small bowel mesentery off of the retroperitoneum (Fig 23-2).
- This dissection is considered complete when the mesentery is mobilized off of the duodenum. It is critical to mobilize the small bowel mesentery to this extent to ensure adequate length of the mesentery to allow the ileal pouch to reach the pelvic floor.

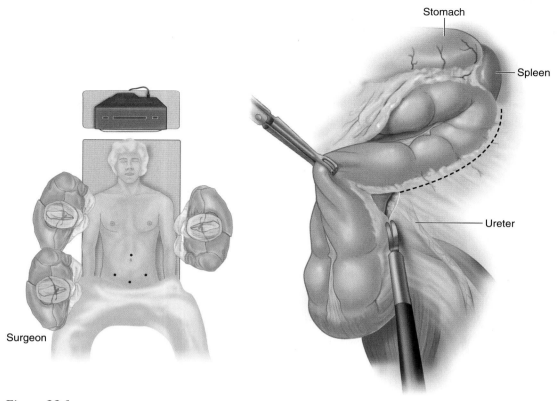

Figure 23-1

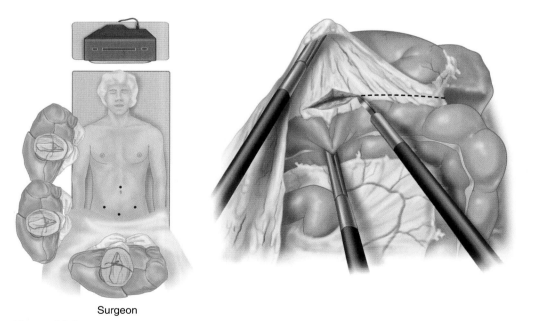

Figure 23-2

- After the small bowel and right colon are mobilized, the hepatic flexure must be freed.
- The patient is repositioned into reverse Trendelenburg maintaining the right side elevated.
- With surgeon and camera operator remaining on the patient's left, the gastro-colic ligament is grasped near the bowel and elevated toward the abdominal wall. Entering the space between the gastro-colic ligament and the transverse mesocolon will facilitate mobilization of the hepatic flexure, which proceeds laterally. (Fig 23-1)
- The duodenum is identified from the superior aspect. With continuous retraction toward the left lower quadrant, the hepatic flexure is freed from the peritoneal attachments to the duodenum and the head of the pancreas.
- Similar to the left colon mobilization of the right colon is only considered complete once the entire right colon and proximal transverse colon can be mobilized to the umbilicus.

Proctectomy

After the colon is fully mobilized, the patient is flattened and returned to maximal Trendelenburg position and the rectal dissection is commenced.

- The surgeon moves to the patient's right side as does the camera operator to begin the dissection. The left pararectal fascia opened after both the left and right ureters are once again identified.
- Scoring the fascia to the left of the rectum, the presacral space is entered. This maneuver is repeated on the right side of the rectum. The surgeon alternates dissecting right to left until the two dissection planes meet behind the rectal

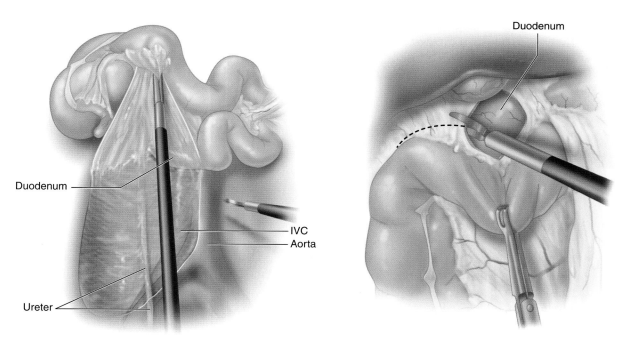

Duodenum

IVC

Aorta

Ureter

Figure 23-3

Duodenum

Figure 23-4

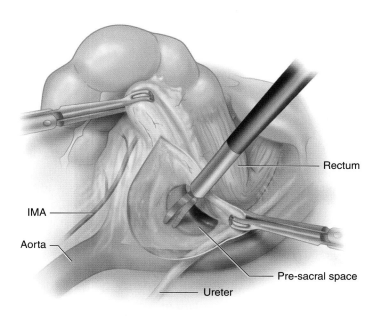

Rectum

IMA

Aorta

Pre-sacral space

Ureter

Figure 23-5

Vessel Ligation

- We routinely use two methods for vessel division.
- In a thin patient, the peri-umbilical extraction site can be used. In this situation, a 4-5 cm peri-umbilical incision is made and the entire colon is exteriorized through this incision. The vessels are then divided extra-corporeally.
- The alternative method is to use a vessel sealing device intra-corporeally.(Fig 23-5) Ideally, this should be a 5 mm instrument to avoid the need for placement of larger trocars.

Exteriorization, Pouch Construction, and Anastomosis

Once all vessels are ligated, the colon and rectum are removed from the abdomen.

- If the vessel were divided via a peri-umbilical incision, this site serves as the extraction site.
- If the vessels were divided intra-corporeally, then a Pfannenstiel incision or a low midline incision may be utilized. The terminal ileum is transected close to the ileal-cecal valve with a linear stapler. The colon specimen is passed off the field and sent to pathology.
- Through the extraction incision, the pouch is constructed extra-corporeally, similar to open surgery. The length is assessed by stretching the small bowel downward externally. If the apex of the proposed pouch reached 3-5 cm below the top of the pubic symphasis, then adequate length is present to perform the anastomosis. If not, then different lengthening maneuvers can be performed.
- The distal ileum is placed in a J configuration and a linear GIA stapler is inserted through an incision at the apex. The lumen of the pouch is constructed by dividing the two opposing internal walls of J-shaped small bowel loop. Usually, two firings of the linear stapler are used to ensure an adequate small bowel reservoir. The anvil of the circular stapler is secured in the pouch apex.
- The pouch is placed back into the abdomen and the extraction site is closed or sealed in a manner that allows pneumoperitoneum to be reestablished.
- The patient is placed in mild Trendelenburg and under laparoscopic visualization an end-to-end anastomosis (EEA) stapler is inserted through the anus and brought out adjacent to the rectal staple line. The anvil exiting the pouch apex is grasped and connected with the rectal EEA stapler.
- Once correct orientation of the pouch and pouch mesentery is confirmed, the stapler is fired. The pelvis is filled with irrigation fluid and under laparoscopic visualization the pouch–anal anastomosis is tested by insufflating the pouch with a proctoscope inserted via the anus.
- A closed suction drain is placed through the left 5-mm ports and positioned behind the pouch.
- A loop ileostomy is constructed approximately 20-25 cm proximal to the pouch and is brought out the site in the right lower quadrant where the 10-12 mm trocar had been placed. The remaining trocars are removed, the fascia and skin incisions are closed, and the loop ileostomy is matured.

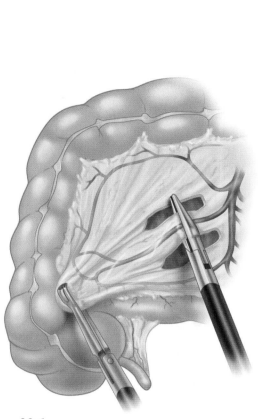

Figure 23-6

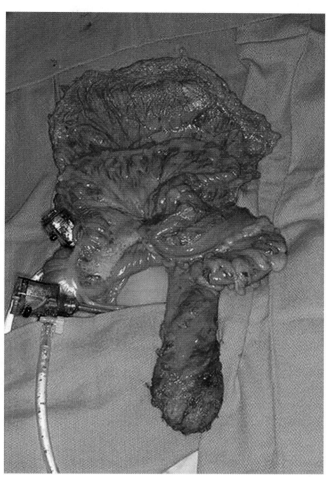

Figure 23-7

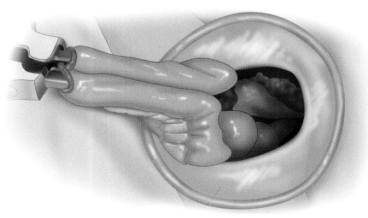

Figure 23-8

Hand-Assisted Approach

The development of special hand-access devices that permit the surgeon to have a hand in the abdomen while maintaining pneumoperitoneum and the ability to use laparoscopic visualization has expanded the number of patients that can have a minimally invasive approach to this complex operation.

- The surgeon can use their hand to retract the colon and to facilitate the dissection. In essence, the hand access device should be considered a "trocar" for the set-up.
- We replace the suprapubic trocar with the hand-access device either using a low midline or Pfannenstiel incision.
- The laparoscopic mobilization of the colon is performed by the surgeon who stands between the patient's legs. The sequence of the colonic mobilization and changes in the patient position during the procedure are the same.
- Since the transverse colon and flexure (hepatic and splenic) vessels may not reach the lower abdomen, intra-corporeal vessel ligation is the norm when using a hand-assisted approach.
- Once the colon is completely mobilized, the rectal dissection can be performed via a laparoscopic approach as previously describe or through the hand-access device using a traditional open approach.
- The pouch can be constructed as previously described and placed down into the pelvis using this incision.

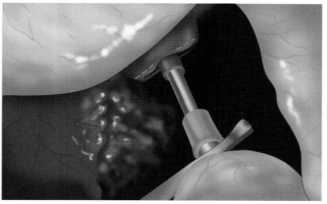

Figure 23-9

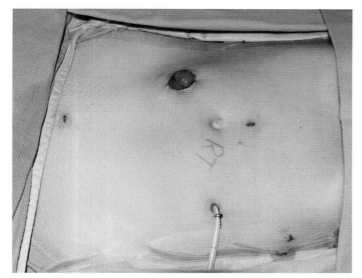

Figure 23-10

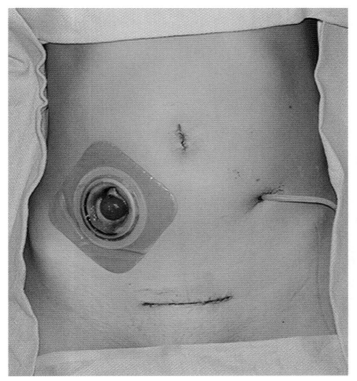

Figure 23-11

Alternative Technical Approach

- Conversion from a laparoscopic approach to an open approach is associated with loss of the short-term clinical benefits of a LA approach and in some studies increased complications. Our practice is to convert from a LA to a HALS approach which retains the short-term benefits of a LA technique.

Step 4. Postoperative Steps

- Only oral gastric tubes are used during the operations and removed at the end of the case.
- IV fluids are minimized during the case and in the post-operative period. Fluid boluses are kept to a minimum as increased total body water is associated with delayed return of bowel function and post-operative complications.
- Urinary catheters are removed 48 hours after surgery.
- All patients are started on a full liquid diet the morning after surgery. This is limited to less than 1 liter intake on the first day. If the full liquids are tolerated, the next day an unrestricted soft diet it begun.

Step 5. Pearls and Pitfalls

A minimally invasive approach to a total proctocolectomy with ileal pouch-anal anastomosis is a technically demanding operation that provides a number of short-term benefits for the patient. Using a systematic approach to the mobilization of the colon and rectum permits a high success rate for completing the procedure laparoscopically. Using a hand-access device is an alternative that may permit a minimally invasive approach for a patient not thought to be a laparoscopic candidate, or to reduce the difficulty of the procedure for a less experienced laparoscopic surgeon.

Selected References

Farouk R, Pemberton JH, Wolff BG, et al. *Functional outcomes after ileal pouch: anal anastomosis for chronic ulcerative colitis.* Ann Surg 231(6):919-26, 2000.

Larson DW, Cima R., *Dozois EJ*, et al: *Safety, feasibility, and short-term outcomes of laparoscopic ileal-pouch anal anastomosis a single institution case-matched experience.* Ann Surg 243(5):667-72, 2006.

Larson DW, Dozois EJ, Piotrowicz K, et al. *Laparoscopic-assisted vs. open ileal pouch–anal anastomosis: functional outcome in a case-matched series.* Dis Colon Rectum 48:1845-50, 2005.

Larson DW, Nelson H. *Laparoscopic colectomy for cancer. J Gastrointest Surg* 8(5):636-42, 2004.

Larson DW, Young-Fadok TM. *Laparoscopic ileal pouch: anal anastomosis.* Rochester, NY, Mayo Clinic, 2002.

Bariatric Surgery

24

ROUX-EN-Y GASTRIC BYPASS (LINEAR STAPLER)

Gordon G. Wisbach and David B. Lautz

Step 1. Surgical Anatomy

- Hepatomegaly—large left lateral segment may require division of falciform ligament for optimal hepatic retraction and visualization of gastric pouch.
- Ligament of Treitz—ensure proper identification by careful manipulation and verification that the small bowel is attached to the retroperitoneum and passes through the transverse mesocolon.
- Where the circular muscular fibers of the esophagus join the oblique fibers of the stomach. Externally, the gastroesophageal fat pad is a consistent identifier of the GE junction.

Step 2. Preoperative Considerations

Patient Preparation

- Bowel preparation consists of a liquid diet the day before surgery.
- Prophylaxis for deep venous thrombosis with sequential compression devices and subcutaneous heparin is started before induction with anesthesia.
- Intravenous cefazolin (or alternatively clindamycin) is administered prophylactically.
- After induction of anesthesia, an orogastric tube and a urinary catheter are placed to decompress the stomach and bladder, respectively.

Equipment and Instrumentation

- ◆ When operating on a morbidly obese patient, it is an obvious and important consideration to have an operating table that is safe for the patient's weight. The table base needs to support the patient's weight plus the weight of foot plates in steep reverse Trendelenburg position without tipping. We prefer a hydraulically operated operating room table that can drop low to the ground, which makes it possible for all surgeons and staff to stand on the ground instead of step stools.
- ◆ An optical trocar is used to access the abdomen once insufflation is obtained with a Veress needle. We prefer this to the open Hassan technique so that we can avoid an umbilical incision, which decreases the risk of hernia formation.
- ◆ A long 45-degree, 10-mm endoscope allows for optimal visualization of the operative anatomy despite variations in body shapes.
- ◆ The expandable liver paddle is easily deployed and offers blunt retraction of the left lobe of the liver, even in very large patients.
- ◆ Additional equipment includes the following:
  - ▲ A suturing device (EndoStitch 10 mm, Covidien, Mansfield, Massachusetts)
  - ▲ A long monopolar L Hook 5 mm (Valley Lab) (ConMed)
  - ▲ Laparoscopic bipolar (LigaSure, Covidien, Mansfield, Massachusetts)
  - ▲ Roticulating laparoscopic staplers (Covidien, Mansfield, Massachusetts)

Anesthesia

- An 18-gauge nasogastric (NG) tube is placed during the creation of the G-J (gastrojejuneal) anastomosis and, as an intraluminal stent, ensures patency.
- A urinary bladder catheter is placed to monitor urinary output.

Room Setup and Patient Positioning

- The patient is placed supine on a well-padded operating table. The arms are extended on padded arm boards and secured with padded straps. Foot plates as well as safety straps on the waist and legs are used to ensure secure positioning, especially during steep reverse Trendelenburg position.
- The operative surgeon stands on the patient's right side while the assistant surgeon and camera operator, if available, are on the patient's left side.
- Monitors are placed at the head of the bed near each shoulder.

Step 3. Operative Steps

Access and Port Placement

- The abdomen is insufflated using a Veress needle in the left upper quadrant. After adequate carbon dioxide pneumoperitoneum to 15 mmHg, an 11-mm optical trocar is advanced in the same quadrant under laparoscopic visualization using a zero-degree scope. A 45-degree laparoscope is then advanced through the Visiport and used to visualize the peritoneal cavity.
- A 10-mm trocar is placed inferolateral to the umbilicus, and the laparoscope is transferred to that position. Two 12-mm and one 5-mm trocars are placed into the right upper quadrant, and a 5-mm trocar is placed lateral to the umbilicus in the left midabdomen (Figure 24-1).

Creation of Jejunojejunostomy (J-J)

- The transverse colon and omentum are retracted superiorly and the ligament of Treitz identified. The proximal jejunum is divided 50 cm from the ligament of Treitz with a linear stapler (2.5 mm). The mesentery between the two limbs of bowel is taken down using the LigaSure device. The proximal jejunum is the pancreaticobiliary limb, containing secretions from remnant stomach as well as liver and pancreas. The distal jejunum will be brought up to the stomach pouch to contain ingested food and is referred to as the Roux limb or alimentary limb.
- The two limbs are joined by a stapled anastomosis after measuring 100 cm distally on the Roux limb. A tacking suture secures the position in preparation for the anastomosis (Figure 24-2).
- Adjoining enterotomies are created. A linear stapler (2.5 mm) is fired distally first (Figure 24-3), then rotated counterclockwise and fired proximally (Figure 24-4). The remaining enterotomy is tacked with 2-0 silks for retraction into a linear stapler (2.5 mm). The enterotomy is closed in a transverse direction to minimize potential narrowing. The small bowel mesenteric defect is closed with a running 2-0 silk suture.
- To prevent obstruction of the biliopancreatic limb (BP) at jejunojejunostomy, we prefer the 180-degree double fire technique.

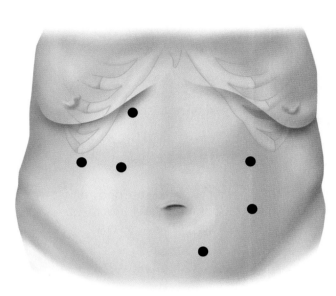

Figure 24-1

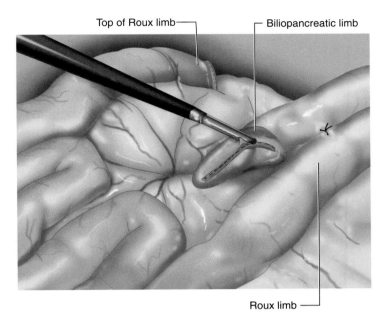

Top of Roux limb

Biliopancreatic limb

Roux limb

Figure 24-2

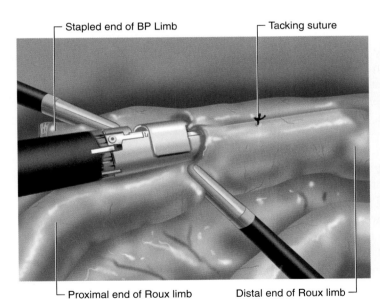

Stapled end of BP Limb

Tacking suture

Proximal end of Roux limb

Distal end of Roux limb

Figure 24-3

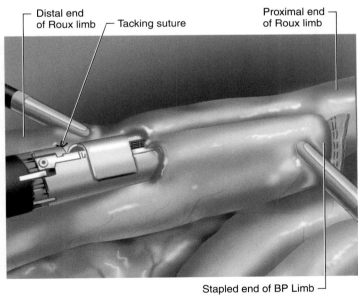

Distal end of Roux limb

Tacking suture

Proximal end of Roux limb

Stapled end of BP Limb

Figure 24-4

Mobilization of Roux Limb to Stomach

- The Petersen space defect, located between the mesentery of the colon and the mesentery of the Roux limb, is closed with a running 2-0 silk, up to the level of the transverse colon (Figure 24-5). By closing the transverse mesocolon onto the retroperitoneum, shortening of the Roux limb mesenteric length is minimized.
- The omentum is inverted over the dome of the liver and then divided from the colon attachment toward the free edge. The fully divided omentum is brought down on either side of the Roux limb.
- Care is taken to ensure no twisting of the Roux limb mesentery when retracted superiorly in an antecolic fashion. This limb is tacked to the anterior wall of the fundus of the stomach to facilitate retrieval during creation of the G-J when the patient is placed in steep reverse Trendelenburg.

Creation of Gastric Pouch

- The patient is placed into the reverse Trendelenburg position. Through a lateral right upper quadrant trocar, an expandable liver paddle is used to retract the left lateral segment of the liver anteriorly off of the stomach, and then the paddle is fixed in position. The location of the GE Junction is determined and at a spot 5 cm distal along the lesser curve of the stomach it is dissected away from the lesser omentum. Through this space dissection is carried into the lesser sac posterior to the stomach, while preserving the vagal trunks (Figure 24-6). The NG tube and esophageal temperature probe are removed from the stomach.
- The pouch of the gastric bypass is created with a series of firings of the linear stapler (3.5 mm). The first firing is with a short stapler straight across the lesser curve followed by a series of firings with a long stapler toward the angle of His. This long staple line is carried parallel to the inferolateral edge of the gastroesophageal fat pad (approximately 1 to 2 cm toward the greater curve of the stomach). Care is taken to place each stapler into the crotch of the previous stapler firing and to ensure that the pouch is completely separated from the gastric remnant. This creates a pouch of approximately 15 mL in size lying along the lesser curve. The transition zones between stapler firings are oversewn with 2-0 silk figure of eight sutures, both along the pouch as well as along the gastric remnant.

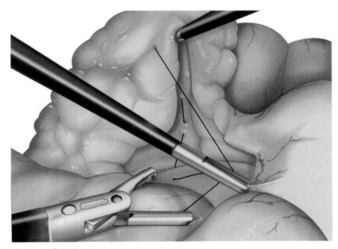

Figure 24-5

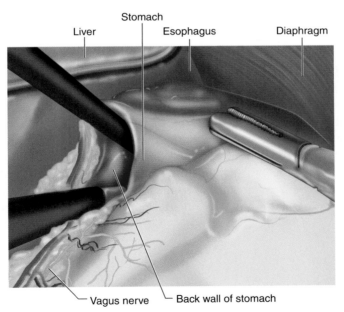

Figure 24-6

Creation of Gastrojejunostomy (G-J)

- The posterior wall of the inferior margin of the pouch is cleared of adhesions and any vascular tissue with the LigaSure device. In preparation for a retrogastric anastomosis, a gastrotomy is created in the posterior wall of the pouch and marked with a silk suture. The stitch previously placed to hold the end of the Roux limb to the fundus is cut and an enterotomy is created approximately 2 cm from the stapled end.
- A 30mm long endoscopic gastrointestinal stapler is used to create the gastrojejunostomy by firing it across the common walls of the posterior pouch and distal Roux limb for approximately 2 cm in length (Figure 24-7). Care is taken to ensure that the gastrojejunostomy is at least 1 cm away from the staple line in the lateral wall of the pouch. Following the staple firing, the anesthesia team places an NG tube and advances it under direct vision across the gastrojejunostomy. The gastrojejunostomy is closed over the NG tube with a running 2-0 silk. This layer is carefully inspected to look for any gaps in the suture line. A second layer of 2-0 silk (running Lembert) is placed circumferentially around the entire anastomosis (Figure 24-8).
- The pouch and the gastrojejunostomy are tested with a methylene blue by clamping the Roux limb, distending the area with blue dye placed through the NG tube, and wrapping the G-J with sponges. Next, an air test is performed by placing the patient in the Trendelenburg position and filling the left upper quadrant with saline. The pouch is distended with air placed through the NG tube while the Roux limb is clamped. The NG tube is advanced forward, and then pulled back into position by the anesthesia team to ensure that it had not been caught by one of the gastrojejunostomy sutures, and securely taped in place.
- The trocars are removed under direct visualization and the pneumoperitoneum is released; 3-0 absorbable suture is used for subcuticular port site closure, and sterile dressings are placed.

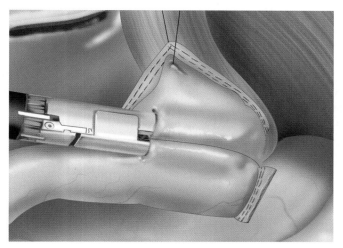

Figure 24-7

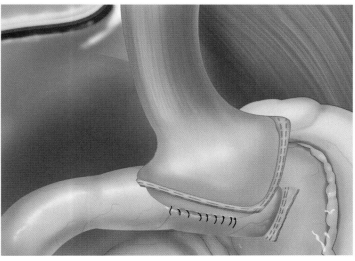

Figure 24-8

Step 4. Postoperative Care

- DVT prophylaxis consists of subcutaneous heparin, bilateral lower extremity pneumatic compression devices while in bed and early ambulation.
- Patients are placed on an aggressive antiemetic regimen.
- The nasogastric tube is placed to gravity drainage and used to stent open the gastrojejunal anastomosis.
- On postoperative day 1, an upper GI is performed before the patient begins a liquid diet. The contrast is first passed through the NG tube to ensure patency. Then the radiologist removes the NG tube, and oral contrast is administered. Often the oral study shows an obstruction at the G-J anastomosis (secondary to the intentionally small anastomosis); however, patients generally tolerate a liquid diet without difficulty. Over the years, we have found that this anastomotic size is the smallest possible without a significant rate of stenosis.
- Oral medication is offered in crushed or elixir form.
- A liquid protein diet is tolerated prior to discharge on the second postoperative day.

Step 5. Pearls and Pitfalls

- *Severity of obesity.* Super obese patients and patients with a long abdomen may require additional port placement. To facilitate creating the J-J anastomosis, an extra 12-mm trocar can be placed to the right and lateral to the umbilicus. As well, long stem trocars may be needed.
- *Long abdomen.* A second camera port can be placed supraumbilically and an additional working port in the right lower quadrant. (see Figure 24-1.)
- *Mobilization of the Roux limb.* Division of the small bowel mesentery to the base usually includes two crossing vascular arcades to ensure adequate length of the Roux limb. Take care to avoid encroachment on the superior mesenteric vessels.

- *BP and Roux limb orientation.* The BP biliopancreatic limb is oriented on the left and toward the end of the Roux limb when creating J-J to prevent BP limb obstruction and allow for closure of Peterson's defect. As well, this orientation will allow preservation of the length of the Roux limb mesentery (the critical length) to facilitate reaching the gastric pouch without tension.
- All mesenteric defects should be closed completely. Although internal hernias are rare, they can be fatal.
- Preserving vagal trunks during the division along the lesser curve when creating the gastric pouch may decrease the incidence of postoperative dysmotility syndrome.
- An 18-gauge NG tube is preferred to stent across G-J during creation of this anastomosis. A smaller diameter tube often curls in the stomach and is difficult to pass.
- Stapler choice—if the patient has a thicker stomach (more common in males), it may be beneficial to use a 4.8-mm (green) load across the antrum; however, in these cases, the 3.5-mm (blue) load should still be used for creation of the G-J.
- Postoperative tachycardia: persistent heart rate greater than 120 bpm for 4 hours mandates further investigation of cause, with a primary focus toward pulmonary embolus or anastomotic leak.

Selected References

Buchwald H, Estok R, Fahrbach K, et al: Weight and type 2 diabetes after bariatric surgery: systemic review and meta-analysis. *Am J Med* 122(3):248-56, 2009.
Kelly JJ, Shikora S, Jones DB, et al: Best practice updates for surgical care in weight loss surgery. *Obesity (Silver Spring)* 17(5): 863-70,2009.
Lehman Center Weight Loss Surgery Expert Panel. Commonwealth of Massachusetts Betsy Lehman Center for Patient Safety and Medical Error Reduction Expert Panel on Weight Loss Surgery: Executive Report update. *Obes Res* 13(2):205-26, 2005.
NIH conference: Gastrointestinal surgery for severe obesity. Consensus Development Conference Panel. *Ann Intern Med* 115(12):956-61, 1991.
Sjo'strom L, Lindroos AK, Peltonen M, et al: Lifestyle, diabetes, and cardiovascular risk factors 10 years after bariatric surgery. *N Engl J Med* 351(26):2683-93, 2004.

25

HANDSEWN GASTROJEJUNAL ANASTOMOSIS

Edward Mun

Step 1. Surgical Anatomy

◆ For pertinent anatomy, see Chapter 24.

Step 2. Preoperative Considerations

◆ For details regarding patient preparation, anesthetic considerations, room set-up & patient positioning, see Chapter 24.

Equipment & Instrumentation

Specialized equipment needed for a hand-sewn gastro-jejunal anastomosis includes:

◆ A needle driver for suturing and a left handed instrument, either a blunt grasper or curved tip grasper.
◆ A large (28 French) gastric evacuation tube, such as Ewald or Mallinkrodt Lavacuator tube (Covidien-Nellcor Products, Boulder, Colorado).

Step 3. Operative Steps

Handsewn Technique.

Access and Port Placement

See Figure 25-1 for port placement reference.

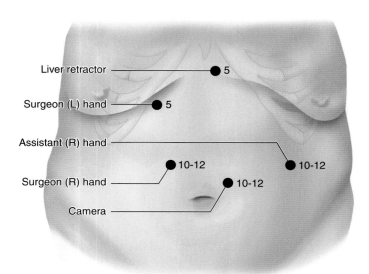

Liver retractor ——————————— ● 5

Surgeon (L) hand ————————— ● 5

Assistant (R) hand ——————————————————— ● 10-12

Surgeon (R) hand ————— ● 10-12

Camera ————————————— ● 10-12

Figure 25-1

Creation of Pouch

♦ For the construction of gastrojejunostomy (following completion of jejunojejunostomy), attention is turned to the upper abdomen for the retraction of the left lobe of the liver. A Nathanson retractor is placed in the epigastrium to elevate the liver, and the gastroesophageal junction is exposed.

♦ The angle of His is mobilized with a Harmonic scalpel.

♦ The pars flaccida of the gastrohepatic ligament is opened. The lesser omentum, located approximately 6 cm from the GE junction, is divided with Harmonic scalpel up to the gastric wall of the lesser curvature.

♦ The stomach is divided transversely using a 45-mm endoscopic gastrointestinal stapler transversely.

♦ This is followed by additional vertical firings of 60 mm Gold cartridges up to the previously mobilized angle of His. A slim gastric pouch (approximately 15 cc's) is created entirely based on the lesser curvature.

Gastrojejunal Anastomosis

♦ The proximal end of the Roux limb is brought to the upper abdomen (usually in an antecolic, antegastric manner).

♦ A running backwall suture line is created using a 2-0 Vicryl suture (~20 cm in length). This is created by lining up the antimesenteric side of the Roux limb to the pouch staple line. The suture is run from the patient's left side corner to the right corner and the remaining suture and needle are saved.

♦ An enterotomy is made into the gastric pouch and the Roux limb (~1 to 1.5 cm in length) a few millimeters away from the running backwall suture line.

♦ An second, inner, running suture line is created using 2-0 Vicryl which is started at the patient's left side corner of the open enterotomy (Figures 25-2, 25-3, and 25-4).

♦ Another 2-0 Vicryl suture is used to close the inner layer anteriorly. Prior to completion of the inner layer closure, a 34 French (1 cm in diameter) large orogastric tube is passed across the anastomosis into the Roux limb to be used as a stent (Figures 25-5).

♦ The inner layer closure is completed by bringing the two sutures onto the anterior aspect of the anastomosis and tying them to each other (Figure 25-6). Needles are cut and removed.

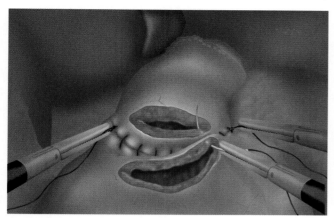

Figure 25-2

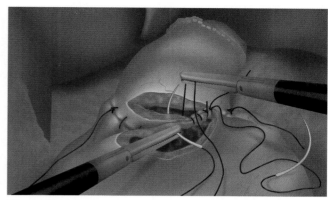

Figure 25-3

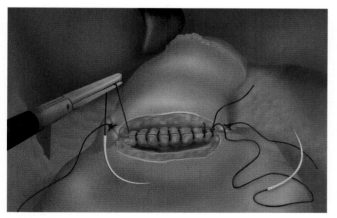

Figure 25-4

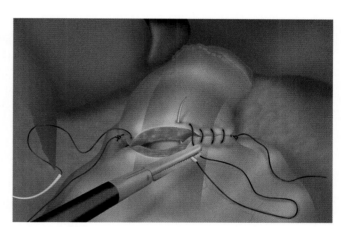

Figure 25-5

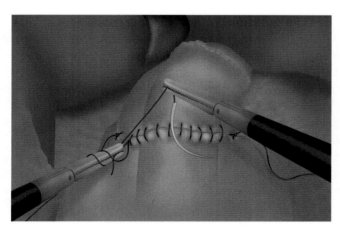

Figure 25-6

- The previous outer layer Vicryl suture is then used to continue anteriorly as Lembert sutures to reinforce the inner layer (Figure 25-7).
- This can be completed by starting a separate second suture beginning from the corner and tying in the middle of the anterior aspect of gastrojejunostomy (Figure 25-8).

Leak Test

- The completed anastomosis is then tested for its integrity. The tip of the Ewald tube is pulled back just beyond the anastomosis, and the Roux limb is occluded with an atraumatic grasper. The patient is placed in the Trendelenburg position, and the left upper quadrant is flooded with normal saline to immerse the anastomosis. Air is introduced into the Roux limb through the tube until adequate inflation of the gastric pouch and proximal Roux limb is observed.
- If leakage (seen as bubbling) is noted, the area is repaired with additional nonabsorbable sutures until no further air leak is noted.

Step 4. Postoperative Care

- A suction drain may be left in the vicinity of this anastomosis for postoperative management.

Step 5. Pearls and Pitfalls

- To minimize the risks of anastomotic ulcers and stricture, at least the inner layer closure is done using absorbable sutures.
- The aperture of the anastomosis is regulated by closing the enterotomy defect over a predetermined caliber bougie or an orogastric tube. Care should be taken to avoid suturing into the tube which can result in disruption of the entire closure.
- Back-hand suturing in the corners may allow more precise suturing if forehand stitching appears awkward in orientation.
- The tension on the running suture is maintained by the assistant throughout the closure process to avoid loosening of the closure and thus, potential anastomotic leakage. Prior to tying the knots, the entire suture is cinched down to further eliminate potential gaps.

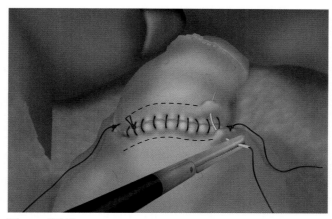

Figure 25-7

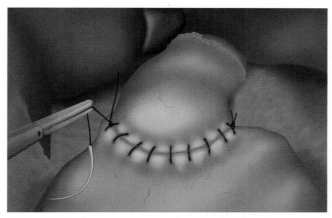

Figure 25-8

26

ADJUSTABLE GASTRIC BANDING

Daniel Davis

Step 1. Surgical Anatomy

- Adjustable gastric banding was first introduced in 1993. Initially the Lap-Band was the only band available, now we have two types: the Lap-Band System by Allergan Health (Figure 26-1) and the Realize Band by Ethicon Endo-Surgery (Figure 26-2).
- The first landmarks to establish are the location of the gastroesophageal junction and the angle of His. Often there will be a large gastroesophageal fat pad, which obscures the location of the gastroesophageal junction. The fat pad will need to be dissected away to identify the gastric serosa.
- Once the gastroesophageal junction is identified, then the presence of a hiatal hernia can be determined. If present, a hiatal hernia will need to be repaired to avoid future dysphagia and failure of the band.
- The hepatogastric ligament, which is part of the lesser omentum, connects the liver with the lesser curve of the stomach. It consists of a caudal flaccid portion known as the "pars flaccida," which is usually transparent and contains no vessels. The right-sided dissection begins here, and there is usually no need to dissect in the more cranial portion of the hepatogastric ligament known as the "pars densa." The pars densa should be avoided when possible because it contains the hepatic branch of the vagus nerve and an associated artery. If there is a replaced left hepatic artery, it will be located in this region and must be considered while dissecting in this region because it is often obscured by overlying fat.
- Once the pars flaccida is opened, the right diaphragmatic crus can be exposed. Proper identification of the right crus is critical to ensure safe dissection into the retrogastric space. Proper technique and placement of band will help the surgeon to avoid entering the lesser sac.
- A perigastric dissection occurs along the lesser curve of the stomach and requires meticulous tissue dissection. This approach may be utilized in cases when there is excess fat along the lesser curve, large accessory or replaced vessels, and poor visibility of the right crus.

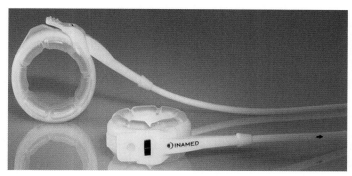

Figure 26-1

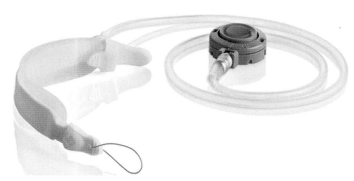

Figure 26-2

Step 2. Preoperative Considerations

Patient Preparation

- The indications and contraindications for an adjustable gastric band are the same for all bariatric surgery patients.
- Preoperative assessment by a multidisciplinary team is required. The team should consist of the following: the bariatric surgeon, internists, endocrinologists, pulmonary staff, and cardiology staff, as well as consultation with nutritionists and psychological evaluation. The assessment is based on the patient's individual needs.
- High body mass index (BMI) >50, advanced age, insulin resistance, and poor health are associated negative predictors but are not contraindications to banding procedures.
- Patients with a history of esophageal disorders or gastroesophageal reflux should undergo an upper GI contrast study, endoscopy and manometry. Any patient with a documented significant esophageal dysmotility disorder should not have a banding procedure.
- Preoperative weight loss is helpful in reducing injury to the liver, reducing operative time, and preparing the patient for postoperative dietary guidelines. Severely obese patients with BMI >50 are recommended to lose >10% of excess weight.

Equipment and Instrumentation

- Three 5-mm bladeless trocars and one 15-mm bladeless trocar (the 15-mm trocar allows safe and easy passage of the band into the abdomen)
- 5-mm 30-degree scope
- Iron Intern with Nathanson liver retractor
- Foot-operated hook cautery for most cases (for patients with excess around the lesser curve and gastroesophageal junction, hand-operated ultrasonic shears are recommended)

Anesthesia

- DVT prophylaxis is recommended in all patients undergoing bariatric surgery. Consensus on mechanical versus pharmacologic versus combination has not been reached. No prospective randomized studies are available. I recommend using a combination of sequential compression devices and 5000 units of unfractionated heparin or 30 mg of low-molecular-weight heparin given subcutaneously 1 hour preoperatively and early ambulation postoperatively.
- Patients with history of DVT and Pulmonary embolism (PE) should be considered for prophylactic vena cava filter as well as patients with pulmonary hypertension, obesity hypoventilation syndrome, and a BMI >60.
- Antiemetics are recommended to reduce vomiting and potential postoperative band prolapse.
- Gastric decompression with NGT or calibration tube will allow easy visualization of anatomic landmarks.

Room Setup and Patient Positioning

- Place the patient in supine or split leg position with foot support, to allow patient to be placed in reverse Trendelenburg for the majority of the procedure.
- Protect all weight-bearing surfaces.
- The surgeon should be on the right side of the patient or between the patient's legs and the assistant should be on the left side.

Step 3. Operative Steps

Access and Port Placement

- Port placement requires five to six ports, one of which should be a bladeless 15-mm port to ease insertion of the band (Figure 26-3).

Exposure and Dissection of Angle of His

- The assistant sweeps greater curvature fat to expose the angle of His, while the surgeon retracts the anterior stomach wall caudally (Figure 26-4).
- Minimal dissection is needed to expose the anterior portion of the left crus.
- Sometimes, greater dissection is needed to identify the esophagogastric junction. The gastro-esophageal fat pad may need to be removed to allow identification of the uppermost stomach, which is necessary for placement of the gastro-gastric sutures later in the procedure. It is best to perform these maneuvers at this stage, while the surgeon still has both hands available.

Exposure of Right Crus and Creation of Retrogastric Tunnel

- Attention is moved to the right of the stomach for creation of the posterior tunnel.
- First, the hepatogastric ligament is opened using electrocautery or ultrasonic energy. Care is taken to avoid injury and bleeding from accessory vessels or a replaced left hepatic artery.
- Once the right crus is identified, we create a small opening at the junction of the right crus and the fatty tissue as far inferior on the crus as possible.
- The blunt-tipped dissecting instrument or grasper will be passed through the opening and into the retrogastric space. There is only a very short distance for the instrument to pass before it is seen exiting at the angle of His (Figure 26-5).
- The tip should pass through the retrogastric tissue without resistance. Any resistance should be worrisome and will require withdrawing the instrument a slight amount and redirecting the tip.

Band Insertion and Positioning

- The band is passed gently through the 15-mm port and directed toward the upper abdomen.
- The tubing of the Lap-Band or the suture of the Realize Band is placed in the tip of the retrogastric instrument. The band is pulled behind the stomach and pulled around the upper portion of the stomach. A 25-cc calibration tube can be used to help position the band if needed.
- The band should sit just below the gastroesophageal junction.
- Prior to buckling, it is important to assess the tightness of the band and remove any excess fat between the band and the stomach, then buckle the band.
- Then we remove the orogastric or calibration tube.
- The band is secured in place by anterior gastro-gastric plicating sutures. These nonabsorbable sutures can be placed in either interrupted or running fashion (Figure 26-6).

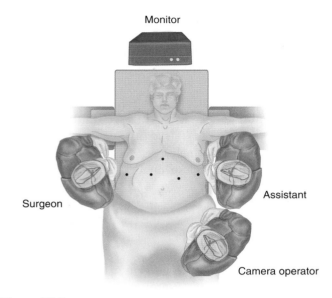

Figure 26-3

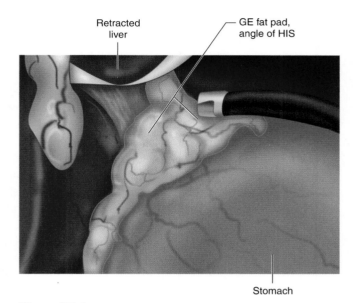

Figure 26-4

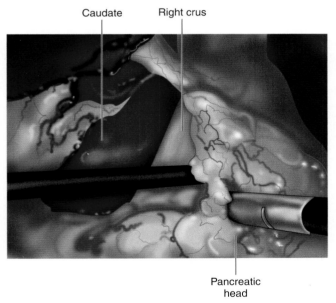

Figure 26-5

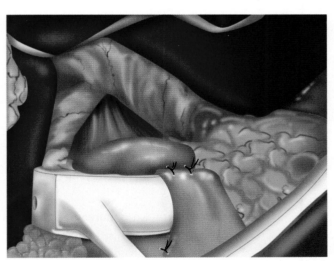

Figure 26-6

Subcutaneous Port Placement

- I have used several techniques over the years:
  - ▲ The most basic method is to extend the incision of the 15-mm port, retract the incision open with narrow Deavers, and place nonabsorbable sutures using handheld instruments into the anterior rectus fascia.
  - ▲ Another technique employed is to place mesh on the port and insert it into the wound. This technique allows a much smaller incision and does not require suturing to the anterior rectus fascia. It is important to create a very small pocket to reduce the risk of port flipping.
  - ▲ Ethicon and Allergan both offer a port applier device to aid with securing the subcutaneous port. The incision is extended and a port applier device is used to secure the port to the fascia.
- The transfascial suture passer technique is the technique I have routinely used for the past few years. This is the same concept that is applied when tacking the four quadrants of mesh in laparoscopic ventral hernia repair using the suture passer.
  - ▲ The port should be placed just lateral to the 15-mm trocar defect.
  - ▲ At end of the case the laparoscope is moved to the most lateral port on the patient's left side. The abdominal wall is visualized laparoscopically visualized where the 15-mm port is located.
  - ▲ The skin incision at the 15-mm port site is only extended enough to allow your finger to sweep the subcutaneous fat away from the fascia while leaving the 15-mm port in place.
  - ▲ Four 0-0 nonabsorbable sutures are placed in a square shape to the right of the 15-mm fascial defect keeping the suture quadrants oriented. This is done using a transfacial suture passer while holding the 15-mm port out of the way. It is important not to include too much peritoneum with each suture bite; this can cause pain with movement.
- The band tubing is pulled out through the 15-mm fascial defect as the port is removed.
- The liver retractor is removed, pneumoperitoneum is released, and all ports are removed.
- The subcutaneous port is attached to the tubing, and the excess tubing is tucked into the abdomen. The subcutaneous port is then parachuted into the wound and secured to the fascia.
- Fascial defects may need to be closed if there is little subcutaneous tissue. Generally, the fascial defect created by the bladeless devices do not require closure especially when located high in the abdomen at the falciform ligament..

Step 4. Postoperative Care

- After surgery, we obtain an esophagram to rule out obstruction/leak and provide a baseline assessment.
- Start clear liquids, and advance to puree for 3 weeks.
- Begin solids at 3 to 4 weeks.
- Office-based adjustments are started 5 weeks after surgery.
- Set a weight-loss goal of 1 to 3 pounds per week.
- Follow up every month or as needed with nutritional counseling.

Step 5. Pearls and Pitfalls

- ◆ Early complications:
- ◆ Gastric perforation related to dissection of angle of His, and passing dissector posterior to stomach.
- ◆ Splenic injury caused by excessive traction on greater curvature fat.
- ◆ Liver injury resulting from a fatty liver.
- ◆ Improper band placement—too high or too low.
- ◆ Avoid postoperative band obstruction by dissecting excessive perigastric fat, removing the gastroesophageal fat pad, and choosing the appropriate size band.
- ◆ Late complications include:
- ◆ Port site infection can be reduced by following proper antiseptic techniques when performing adjustments. If port site infection occurs, a trial of oral antibiotics is recommended. If the patient does not improve, it will be necessary to rule out band erosion with upper endoscopy.
- ◆ Band prolapse occurs approximately 5% to 10% of the time and requires reoperation to reposition or replace band.
- ◆ Band erosion occurs in 1% to 2% of patients. Avoid excessive traction on stomach and do not cover buckle area of band with stomach to reduce erosion. If erosion is diagnosed, the band will have to be removed.
- ◆ Esophageal dilatation occurs approximately 5% of the time, because of over-tightening of the band and poor follow-up. It is recommended to deflate the band for 1 month and repeat the esophagram. Once the esophagus diameter has improved, the surgeon may readjust.

Selected References

Belachew M, Legrand M, Vincenti VV, et al: *Laparoscopic placement of adjustable silicone gastric band in the treatment of morbid obesity: how to do it.* Obes Surg 5(1):66-70, 1995.

O'Brien PE, Dixon JB: *Laparoscopic adjustable gastric banding.* In Inabnet WB, DeMaria EJ, Ikramuddin S (editors): *Laparoscopic Bariatric Surgery,* Lippincott Williams & Wilkins, Melbourne, Australia, 2005, pp. 75-84.

Vertruyen M: *Experience with Lap-Band System up to 7 years.* Obes Surg 12(4):569-72, 2002.

27

COMPLICATIONS OF ADJUSTABLE GASTRIC BANDING

Emma Patterson and Mark Smith

Step 1. Surgical Anatomy

- Band complications can occur early or late. The most common late complications are port or tubing problems (2% to 3%), band slippage (3% to 6%), and band erosion (0.5% to 1%). We will concentrate on band slippage and band erosion in this chapter.
- In revisional operations, caution should be paid to the left gastric artery, or an aberrant left hepatic artery arising from the left gastric. These relatively large vessels can be obscured by a dense inflammatory reaction and may be unrecognized when dissecting to the left of the stomach and band buckle.
- The operative treatment of band slippage involves laparoscopic reduction of the herniated stomach, with band replacement or repositioning. This is usually possible via a laparoscopic approach. Contrast swallow shows an eccentric pouch enlargement above the band and that the angle of the band to the vertical is greater than 90 degrees (Figure 27-1 and 27-2).
- A hiatal hernia is commonly found in association with a band slip and should be repaired at the time of revisional surgery. Exploration reveals a dilated, eccentric gastric pouch above the band (Figure 27-2).

Step 2. Preoperative Considerations

Patient Preparation

- The modern technique of band placement is the pars flaccida approach, favored because of a decreased incidence of posterior band slippage. There is minimal posterior dissection at the level of the confluence of the left and right diaphragmatic crura. The posterior position of the band is at or just below the esophagogastric junction. Anteriorly a small (15 mL) virtual pouch is created.

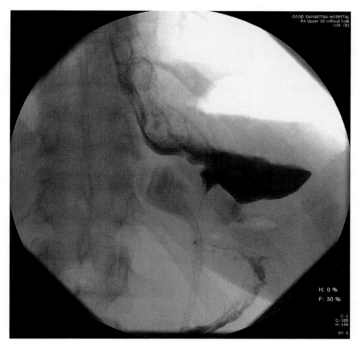

Figure 27-1

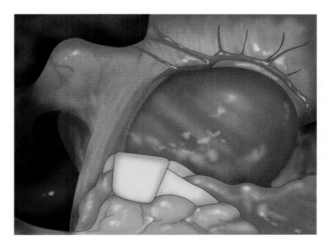

Figure 27-2

- All patients should have a reassessment of their comorbidities and nutritional state before undergoing revisional bariatric surgery. Patients may develop anemia after band slippage secondary to erosive gastritis in the dilated pouch.
- Diagnosis and anatomy should be well defined preoperatively; the investigation of choice for band slip is a contrast swallow, and for band erosion it is an upper endoscopy.

Equipment and Instrumentation

- We perform the procedure with a 10-mm, 30-degree angled laparoscope.
- Long instruments are routinely used.
- Spatula cautery is preferred, and electrosonic coagulation is not necessary.
- A Nathanson retractor is used for liver retraction.

Anesthesia

- Strict attention should be paid to venous thromboembolism prophylaxis and antibiotic prophylaxis.

Room Setup and Patient Positioning

- The patient is positioned supine on the operating table with the arms abducted and the legs together.

Step 3. Operative Steps

Access and Port Placement

- Trocar placement is similar to primary laparoscopic adjustable gastric banding.
- Care should be taken to avoid the existing access port, which can be retained for use with the new band.

For Band Slippage

- Initial dissection using cautery should proceed along the band tubing with sequential division of biomembrane until the band is reached.
- The band must be dissected away from biomembrane, adhesions, and the left lateral section of the liver until the buckle is free.
- After the buckle of the band is free, the band may be cut with hook scissors (Figure 27-3). Retaining the band for use as a retractor during some of the remaining dissection may also be useful.

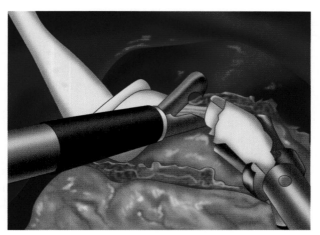

Figure 27-3

- The previous tunnel formed by the gastro-gastric sutures is usually taken down. This can be achieved through careful dissection using laparoscopic scissors. If the dissection plane is not clear, a linear cutting stapler may be used to avoid inadvertent gastrotomy.
- Crural defects should be repaired prior to placement of a new band. I close anteriorly (Figure 27-4) or posteriorly (Figures 27-5A and 27-5B), and sometimes both, wherever I find the gap.
- We then replace the band using a new adjustable gastric band placed via the pars flaccida technique posteriorly and in a higher position anteriorly.
- Gastro-gastric sutures are placed between fundus and gastric pouch anteriorly to prevent reslip. Occasionally I will omit sutures on revisions as they place too much tension.
- An EndoCatch (Covidien, Mansfield, Massachusetts) bag facilitates removal of the old band.
- The tip of the tubing of the new band is brought out and spliced to the existing access port extracorporeally using a metal connector that comes with the new band.

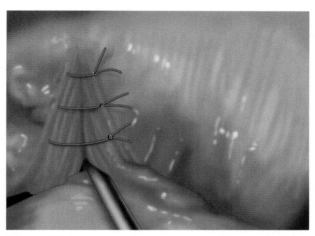

Figure 27-4

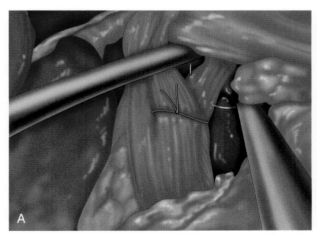

Figure 27-5 A

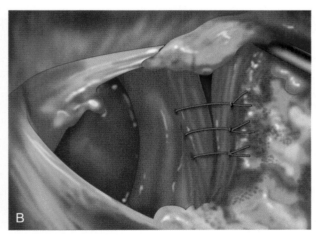

Figure 27-5 B

For Band Erosion

- An adjustable gastric band can be seen with a retroflexed endoscope. It is eroding into stomach lumen (Figure 27-6).
- The treatment of band erosion involves band removal, via an endoscopic, or laparoscopic approach, along with closure of the gastric perforation. We favor the latter technique as it facilitates the gastric repair.
- Patient positioning and trocar placement is as for band slippage.
- Initial dissection is with electrocautery, using the tubing to identify the position of the band if possible.
- The buckle of the band is dissected free, and the band is cut with hook scissors.
- The band is then removed, and the gastric perforation then repaired using laparoscopically placed sutures in two layers (Figures 27-7 and 27-8).
- Gastric integrity is tested using methylene blue dye, and fibrin glue is applied.
- A closed low suction drain is sometimes placed adjacent to the gastrotomy closure.

Step 4. Postoperative Care

- Band repositioning or replacement is usually done as an outpatient procedure, whereas band removal for erosion may spend a night.
- We usually admit patients to the ward for overnight observation following revisional laparoscopic adjustable gastric band surgery.
- Patients are usually kept NPO until after a water soluble contrast swallow on postoperative day.
- Oral fluids are then commenced at a rate of 30 mL every 15 minutes.
- Patients are discharged when they can tolerate 240 mL of fluid orally over a period of 2 hours.
- Patients follow a liquid diet for 2 weeks and a puree diet for 2 weeks. The first band adjustment is usually performed at 4 weeks after the operation.
- For band erosion, further revisional surgery is considered after full recovery from band removal. Options include re-gastric banding, Roux-en-Y gastric bypass, and sleeve gastrectomy.

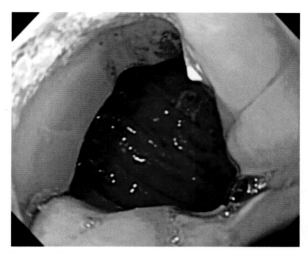

Figure 27-6

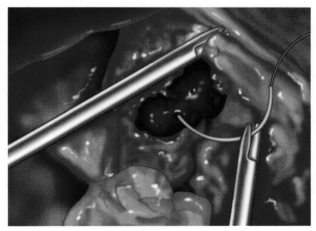

Figure 27-7

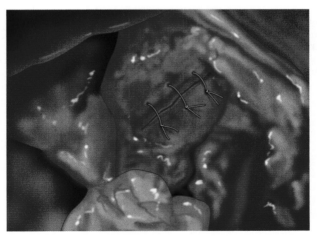

Figure 27-8

Step 5. Pearls and Pitfalls

- In an erosion, because of the dense inflammatory reaction, the tubing may not be visible; if this is the case, then dissection should start underneath the left lateral section of the liver. The tubing will be found adherent to the liver in this location and may then be followed to the band.
- When dense adhesions make dissecting out an eroded gastric band extremely hazardous, an alternative approach is to remove it transgastrically via a distal gastrotomy, as long as the buckle is within the stomach. A combined laparoscopic/endoscopic approach is also possible in this situation.
- Care should be taken to avoid an accessory left hepatic artery running in the gastrohepatic omentum when dissecting out the gastric band. This is especially true for band erosion.
- It is important to repair any hiatal hernia or crural weakness found in association with a band slip. This can be repaired using sutures placed anterior or posterior to the esophagus.
- When replacing a gastric band after a slip, sutures from the greater curve to the lesser curve below the band, imbricating the redundant fundus, may help to prevent reslippage.
- When further revisional surgery is contemplated, such as after band erosion, adhesion prevention barriers, such as SurgiWrap (Mast Biosurgery, Zurich, Switzerland), will facilitate subsequent dissections.

Selected References

Chevallier JM, Zinzindohoue F, Douard R, et al: Complications after laparoscopic adjustable gastric banding for morbid obesity: experience with 1,000 patients over 7 years. *Obes Surg* 14(3):407-14, 2004.
Cunneen SA, Phillips E, Fielding G, et al: Studies of Swedish adjustable gastric band and Lap-Band: systematic review and meta-analysis. *Surg Obes Relat Dis* 4(2):174-85, 2008.
Mehanna MJ, Birjawi G, Moukaddam HA, et al: Complications of adjustable gastric banding, a radiological pictorial review. *AJR Am J Roentgenol* 186(2):522-34, 2006.
Ponce J, Fromm R, Paynter S, et al: Outcomes after laparoscopic adjustable gastric band repositioning for slippage or pouch dilation. *Surg Obes Relat Dis* 2(6):627-31, 2006.

28

SLEEVE GASTRECTOMY

Gregory F. Dakin and Alfons Pomp

Step 1. Surgical Anatomy

- ◆ The stomach has a rich blood supply, which includes the left and right gastric arteries, the left and right gastroepiploic arteries, and the short gastric vessels. This operation involves removal of the majority of the stomach, leaving behind a narrow "sleeve" of stomach based along the lesser curvature, with vascularization essentially derived from the left gastric artery. The vagus nerves on the lesser curve of the stomach are left intact.
- ◆ Special consideration is given at the angle of His to ensure the entire left diaphragmatic crus is freed from attachments, such that transection of the stomach does not leave a posterior pouch of fundus on the proximal portion of the sleeve. Reduction of hiatal hernia may be necessary to ensure complete removal of redundant fundus.

Step 2. Preoperative Considerations

Patient Preparation

- ◆ Sleeve gastrectomy may be performed on those patients who qualify for bariatric surgery (i.e., meet National Institutes of Health (NIH) criteria and have satisfied a multidisciplinary evaluation by a weight-loss surgery team). This operation has been generally offered as an "initial stage" in patients who are at high risk for other more traditional bariatric operations. Sleeve gastrectomy is considered for the following high-risk patients:
  - ▲ Any patient with a body mass index (BMI) >60 kg/m^2
  - ▲ Patients with android body habitus
  - ▲ Patients with significant previous intestinal surgery
  - ▲ Patients with cirrhosis or esophageal/gastric varices (severe hepatic disease may preclude all types of weight loss surgery)
  - ▲ Patients with inflammatory bowel disease
  - ▲ Patients who have had chronic NSAID use
- ◆ After significant weight loss, these patients may undergo a "second-stage" operation with conversion to either Roux-en-Y gastric bypass or biliopancreatic diversion with duodenal

switch. With excellent initial weight loss results and increasing experience with the operation, many groups are now offering it as a stand-alone procedure in average-risk patients.

◆ Special attention in the history and physical should elicit any signs of liver disease and cirrhosis. In diabetic patients, if there is a clinical suspicion of gastroparesis, gastric emptying studies should be considered. Preoperative upper endoscopy should be performed to diagnose hiatal hernia and rule out gastric lesions or helicobacter pylori infection.

Equipment and Instrumentation

◆ Standard laparoscopic instruments are used throughout the case. Depending on the type of stapler used, 15-mm disposable trocars may be necessary. We commonly use a buttress material on the stapler cartridges to aid in hemostasis. Either ultrasonic energy or LigaSure (Covidien, Mansfield, Massachusetts) can be used for division of the vascular attachments.

Anesthesia

◆ A team experienced with the morbidly obese population should administer general anesthesia. These patients often have extremely difficult airways and may require a full complement of adjunctive airway techniques, including awake fiberoptic intubation.

Patient Positioning

◆ The patient is best positioned supine with both arms abducted and the legs split. The surgeon stands between the legs with an assistant holding the camera on the patient's right and an additional assistant on the left.
◆ The patient is placed in reverse Trendelenburg position throughout the procedure.

Step 3. Operative Steps

Access and Port Placement

◆ Pneumoperitoneum can be established via a variety of time-honored techniques.
◆ Trocars are placed as follows: a 15-mm trocar at the umbilicus, a 5-mm trocar in the right upper quadrant, 5-mm trocar in the epigastrium, a 5-mm trocar in the left upper quadrant, and a 5-mm trocar in the lateral left upper quadrant. The Nathanson liver retractor is placed via an additional 5-mm incision in the high-epigastrium. Alternatively, trocars can be placed in the right and left upper quadrant for use in stapling (Figure 28-1).

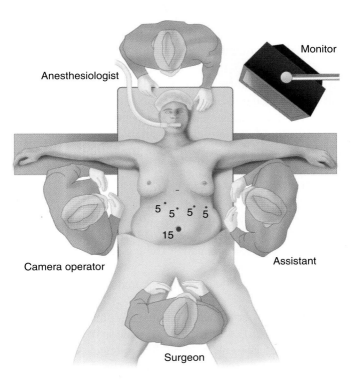

Figure 28-1

Operative Steps

- The gastrocolic omentum is divided off the greater curvature of the stomach, beginning approximately 5 cm proximal to the pylorus and proceeding to the angle of His. The entire fundus is freed posteriorly from the left crus. Posterior attachments to the pancreas are also divided such that the stomach is only attached via its lesser curvature blood supply (Figure 28-2).
- If present, a hiatal hernia should be reduced. A large gastric fat pad can be resected.
- Transection of the stomach begins on the antrum 5 cm proximal to the pylorus with a 60-mm long, 4.8-mm articulating stapler. The 4.8-mm stapler can be used for the entire resection with the addition of commercially available buttress materials. Alternatively, staples that are 3.5 mm in height can be used in the thinner, more proximal portions of the stomach.
- The transection is oriented along the lesser curvature such that the stomach is not narrowed at the incisura (Figure 28-3).
- After two staple firings, a 40 F bougie is placed by the anesthesia team and directed toward the pylorus along the lesser curvature. The remainder of the stomach transection is performed while pushing the bougie against the lesser curvature to guide the resection as it proceeds toward the angle of His.
- The staple line is closely inspected, and portions may be oversewn to ensure hemostasis as necessary.
- A methylene blue leak test is performed. The distal stomach is occluded with a bowel grasper while approximately 60 cc of methylene blue is instilled under gentle pressure created with a bulb syringe. The entire staple line is checked not only for leaks but for proper formation of the staples, particularly around the thick antrum (Figure 28-4).
- The specimen is removed using a bag via the 15-mm umbilical trocar. The umbilical port can be stretched with a large clamp prior to extraction. The incision generally does not need to be lengthened significantly if the stomach specimen is placed in the bag with the distal (antral) portion of the staple line protruding out. This enables the staple line to be grasped and the stomach delivered from the bag, rather than blindly grabbing the larger fundic portion.

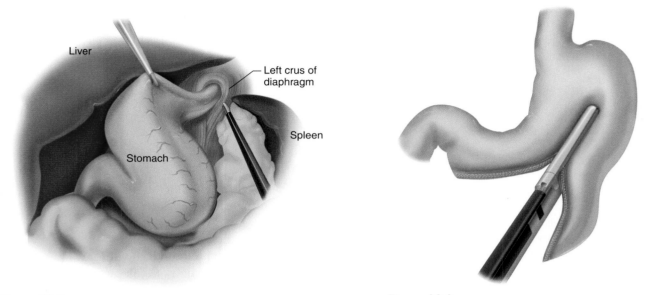

Figure 28-2

Figure 28-3

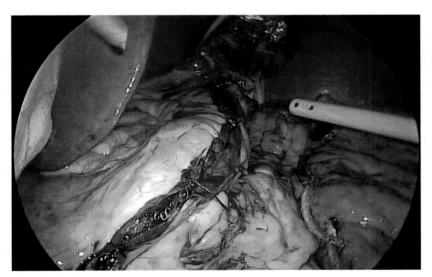

Figure 28-4

Step 4. Postoperative Care

- ◆ Patients are monitored in an appropriate setting before transfer to the floor.
- ◆ An upper gastrointestinal series may be obtained on the first postoperative day to exclude leaks and evaluate gastric function and anatomy (Figure 28-5).
- ◆ Diet is liquids on the first day, and it progresses to pureed food on the second day. Patients are usually discharged home on the second postoperative day.

Step 5. Pearls and Pitfalls

- ◆ Staple the antrum with caution, as this tissue may be relatively thick and could cause stapler misfire or fracturing of the tissue. If staple line reinforcement products are used, it may be prudent to forego them in the antral area.
- ◆ It is extremely important to have the anesthesiologist hold the bougie in place throughout the entire resection of the stomach. Failure to do so may result in an unnoticed withdrawal of the bougie away from the lesser curvature and inadvertent transection of the bougie or the stomach.
- ◆ The final staple firing should veer away from the gastroesophageal junction so that the esophagus is avoided. The thinner esophageal wall and absence of serosa make it vulnerable to inadequate stapler closure, which may contribute to leak formation.
- ◆ Carefully inspect the entire gastric staple line upon completion to ensure all staples are well formed and oversew portions as necessary, especially at the junction of stapler firings.
- ◆ Patients may experience significant reflux, nausea, and dysphagia, which can be managed with appropriate medications postoperatively.

Selected References

Moy J, Pomp A, Dakin G, et al: Laparoscopic sleeve gastrectomy for morbid obesity. *Am J Surg* 196(5):e56-e59, 2008.

Lee CM, Cirangle PT, Jossart GH: Vertical gastrectomy for morbid obesity in 216 patients: report of two-year results. *Surg Endosc* 21(10):1810-16, 2007.

Lalor PF, Tucker ON, Szomstein S, Rosenthal RJ: Complications after laparoscopic sleeve gastrectomy. Surg Obes Relat Dis 4(1):33-38, 2008.

Parikh M, Gagner M, Heacock L, et al: Laparoscopic sleeve gastrectomy: does bougie size affect mean %EWL? Short-term outcomes. *Surg Obes Relat Dis* 4(4):528-33, 2008.

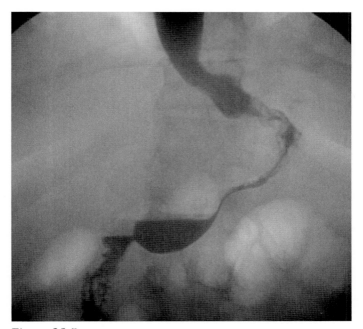

Figure 28-5

INDEX

Positioning and setup
for abdominal washout, 84
for adrenalectomy, 146
for appendectomy, 205f, 206
for cholecystectomy, 89, 92
for component separation (abdominal wall), 182
for cystgastrostomy, transgastric, 108
for esophagectomy, 13, 15f
for gastric banding, adjustable, 280
for gastric wedge resection, 64, 65f
for Heller myotomy fundoplication for achalasia, 28, 29f
lateral decubitus position, 117
for left colon resection (medial to lateral approach), 232
for left lateral sectionectomy, 98, 99f
for Nissen fundoplication, 39
padded cradle "airplane" position, 117
for pancreatectomy, distal, 117, 119f
for pancreaticojejunostomy, 130
for paraesophageal hernia, 51
for peptic ulcer surgery, 73
for proctocolectomy, total (ileal-pouch anal anastomosis), 241, 242
for right colectomy, hand-assisted, 216, 219f
for right hemicolectomy, 225
for Roux-en-Y gastric bypass (linear stapler), 255
for sleeve gastrectomy, 288
for splenectomy, 139
for ventral incisional herniorrhaphy, 169
for Zenker's diverticulum, 6
Pouch construction, 246, 247f
Preperitoneal space, 159-162, 161f
Proctectomy, 244-246, 245f, 247f
Proctocolectomy, total (ileal-pouch anal anastomosis), 239-250
anesthesia for, 240
dissection in, 242-246, 243f, 245f, 247f
emergent versus elective, 239
equipment and instrumentation for, 240
exteriorization and pouch construction in, 246-248, 247f
hand-assisted approach, 248
indications for, 239
port placement in, 241, 243f
positioning and setup for, 241, 242
postoperative care in, 250
preoperative considerations in, 240-241
specific considerations in, 239, 250
surgical anatomy for, 239
Prophylaxis. *See also* Antibiotics, prophylactic.
before adrenalectomy, 146
before appendectomy, 201
before bariatric surgery, 253
before component separation (abdominal wall), 182
against deep vein thrombosis, 89, 116, 138, 216, 225
before peritoneal dialysis catheter placement, 190
before splenectomy, 137, 138
before ventral incisional herniorrhaphy, 168
Proton pump inhibitors (PPIs), 71, 83
Pulmonary function tests, 50
Pulorus, 78
Pyloroplasty, 24, 25f, 76
Pylorus, 71

Q

Quinton percutaneous insertion kit, 196

R

Realize Band by Ethicon Endo-surgery, 270, 271f, 276
Rectum
dissection of, 236, 237f
location of, 245f
Rectus abdominis muscle, 157f, 161f, 178, 179f, 188
Renin level, 144
Retained antrum, 78
Right colectomy, hand-assisted, 212-222
anesthesia for, 216
diagnostic imaging for, 215
dissection in, 218
equipment and instrumentation for, 215
port placement in, 216, 219f
positioning and setup for, 216, 219f
postoperative care in, 220
preoperative considerations in, 214-216
specific considerations in, 214, 221-222
surgical anatomy for, 212-214
Right crus, 270, 274, 275f
Right hemicolectomy, 223-230
anastomoses in, 228
anesthesia for, 225
contraindications to, 223
dissection in, 226, 228
equipment and instrumentation for, 224
indications for, 223
port placement in, 225, 226, 227f
positioning and setup for, 225
postoperative care in, 230
preoperative considerations in, 223-225
surgical anatomy for, 223
Right lower quadrant (RLQ), 201, 206
Round ligament (ligamentum teres), 97, 101f
Roux limb (alimentary limb), 19f, 134, 135f, 256, 257f, 262, 266-268
Roux-en-Y gastric bypass (linear stapler), 251-263
anesthesia for, 255
diagnostic imaging for, 262
equipment and instrumentation for, 254
gastric pouch creation in, 258
gastrojejunostomy creation in, 260
jejunojejunostomy creation in, 256
limb creation in, 256, 257f, 258
port placement for, 256, 257f
positioning and setup for, 255
postoperative care in, 262
preoperative considerations in, 253-255
safety precautions in, 254, 255
specific considerations in, 262-263
surgical anatomy for, 253

S

Sacral promontory, 233f
Sequential compression devices (SCDs), 138, 168
Sigmoid colon, 233f
Skin
marking of, 171f, 214, 215
release by undermining, 174, 175f
Sleeve gastrectomy, 287-293
anesthesia for, 288
diagnostic imaging for, 288, 292, 293f
dissection in, 290, 291f
equipment and instrumentation for, 288
indications for, 287-288
port placement for, 288, 289f
positioning and setup for, 288
postoperative care in, 292
preoperative considerations in, 287-288
specific considerations in, 292
specimen removal in, 290
surgical anatomy for, 287

Sling fibers of Willis, 27, 30, 31f, 36, 37f
Smoking, 83
Solid organ surgery
cystgastrostomy, transgastric, 105-114
laparoscopic pancreatico-jejunostomy (Puestow procedure),
pancreatectomy, 115-127
splenectomy, 137-142
Specimen retrieval bags. *See* EndoCatch bag.
Specimens
morcellation of, 140, 142
removal of, 228, 247f, 290
Spermatic cord, 165f
Spleen
accessory, 142
preservation of, 124, 125f
procedure for removal, 140
size of, 137
Splenectomy, 137-142
anesthesia for, 138
diagnostic imaging for, 137, 138
equipment and instrumentation for, 138
port placement in, 139-142, 141f
positioning patient for, 139
postoperative care in, 142
preoperative considerations in, 137-139
specific considerations in, 142
surgical anatomy for, 137
Splenic artery, 107, 122, 123f, 124, 125f, 127
Splenic flexure, 120-122, 140, 150, 151f, 236, 237f, 238
Splenic vein, 122, 123f, 124, 125f, 127
Splenocolic ligament, 120, 121f, 140, 141f
Splenophrenic ligament, 140
Splenorenal ligament, 152
Spot size, 8
Staging of cancer, 214, 218, 223
Stapler technique, 100, 101f, 104, 122, 256, 257f, 258, 292
Stapling devices. *See* GIA endostaplers.
Stents, pancreatic, 128, 132
Steroid hormones, 143
Steroids
prophylactic, 137
stress dose of, 146, 154
Stoma sites, 240
Stomach
figures of, 15f, 17f, 67f
irrigation of, 84
mobilization of, 66
resection of, 68
retraction of, 131, 133f
Stone extraction, 132
Subcutaneous tunnel, 194, 195f
Suction irrigator, 206
Surgiwrap by Mast Biosurgery, 286
Suture materials
for appendectomy, 208
for gastrojejunostomy, 261f
management of, 86
for mesh fixation, 172, 173f
Swan neck presternal catheter, 196

T

Tachycardia, 263
Taenia coli, 208
Tattoos, 213f, 214, 215, 223, 238
Terminal ileum, 208, 209f
Thrombocytopenia, 138
Tissue sealant, 124
Toradol, 220